Namir Katkhouda

Namir Katkhouda

Advanced Laparoscopic Surgery

Techniques and Tips

2nd Edition

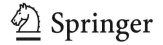 Springer

Namir Katkhouda, MD
Professor of Surgery
Vice Chairman for Clinical Affairs
Chief, Division of General and
Laparoscopic Surgery
Director, Bariatric Surgery Program
University of Southern California
Keck School of Medicine
Department of Surgery
1510 San Pablo St.
Los Angeles, CA 90033, USA
katkhoud@surgery.usc.edu or nkatkhouda@surgery.usc.edu

Illustrator:
Timothy C. Hengst
1631 Calle de Oro
Thousand Oaks
CA 91360-7012, USA
tim@thengst.com

ISBN 978-3-540-74842-7   eISBN 978-3-540-74843-4

Springer Heidelberg Dordrecht London New York

Library of Congress Control Number: 2010935945

© 1998 W.B. Saunders Company Ltd., 2010 Springer-Verlag Berlin Heidelberg

Cover design: eStudio Calamar, Figueres/Berlin

Printed on acid-free paper

Springer is part of Springer Science+Business Media (www.springer.com)

To God, who guides my life.

To my wife, Dominique, for her eternal love and support.

Without her, many important things would not have happened.

To my beloved children, Nadine and Philippe.

They deserve the absolute best for their understanding of their "busy" father.

To my mother whom I love dearly.

To my brothers.

In memory of my father.

Preface

When I wrote and published the first edition of Advanced Laparoscopic Surgery "Techniques and Tips" in 1998, I wanted to share with all general surgeons, residents, attendings and senior faculty alike the experience that I accumulated in laparoscopic surgery over a period of 10 years. I knew at the time that the biggest hurdles for a wide adoption of advanced techniques were the specialized surgical skills involved, including laparoscopic suturing. The chapters included the procedures that were performed routinely and for which there was evidence to support the practice of the techniques. The continued success of the book after it was translated into Spanish and its widespread sale even in Asia confirmed that I was correct in my assumptions. My greatest satisfaction was that the "red book", as it became known, was on the shelf of most surgical residency program libraries. In 2008, 10 years later and 20 years following my first laparoscopic cholecystectomy, I embarked on another big project, namely to write the second edition. For this book, I deleted procedures that were abandoned, such as laparoscopic spine fusion, but added all the newest procedures, including laparoscopic ventral hernia repair, laparoscopic hepatectomy, and a large chapter on laparoscopic bariatric surgery including gastric bypass, gastric band and sleeve gastrectomy. I also ensured that the newest, most innovative techniques were presented, such as laparoscopic single access surgery, and of course advanced laparoscopic suturing , the Holy Grail of advanced laparoscopic surgery, a skill without which advanced laparoscopic training remains incomplete.

I did not forget the rest of the GI procedures, many of which were redone, and color figures were added. Another new feature is the inclusion of 2 DVDs of some of my techniques so readers can get a more "live" idea of my concepts.

I hope that I have reached the ambitious goals that I set forth in this "blue book": complex laparoscopic techniques made simpler and upheld by surgical excellence.

Los Angeles, February 14, 2010   NAMIR KATKHOUDA, MD, FACS

Acknowledgements

ASHKAN MOAZZEZ, MD
Assistant Professor of Clinical Surgery
Division of General and Laparoscopic Surgery
Department of Surgery
University of Southern California

His assistance was invaluable

TIM HENGST
Medical illustrator

His artistic talent is unsurpassed

VAUGHN A. STARNES, MD, FACS
Distinguished Professor and Chairman
Department of Surgery
Founder and Director, USC Cardiothoracic Institute
University of Southern California

"In the USC Department of Surgery", he once said, "surgical excellence is
minimum standard". I could not agree more. For his confidence and friendship.

Contents

11 INCISIONAL AND VENTRAL HERNIA REPAIR INCLUDING COMPONENT SEPARATION

12 SPLENECTOMY (TOTAL AND PARTIAL) AND SPLENOPANCREATECTOMY

General Concepts 1

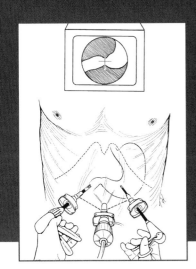

Before commencing any laparoscopic procedure it is of paramount importance to go through a checklist to ensure the working environment is as comfortable as possible. Working from monitors creates an unnatural and abstract environment that requires manual skill, concentration, and coordination of hands and brain; hence it is crucial that the surgeon be comfortable to allow optimum technical performance.

The Checklist Approach

The Team

A successful laparoscopic program is dependent on harmonious interaction within the surgical team. Whenever possible the nursing staff should be dedicated to the laparoscopic surgical program. Only then they will be able to excel in all aspects of the procedure, both technical and medical. The circulating nurse should work in harmony with the scrub technician and both should observe procedures carefully to allow them to anticipate problems and preempt the surgeon's requests. This also requires knowledge of the instruments, their functions, and construction in order to replace or repair instruments when necessary.

It is also important that both the scrub technician and the circulating nurse have a basic knowledge of video imaging to be able to connect and disconnect TV monitors and video recorders, and to assist if problems arise with the imaging system. In the ideally staffed operating theater, a third dedicated technical support person is responsible for maintenance of the sophisticated electronic equipment.

The team is created by selecting committed individuals from the surgical staff, teaching them the basic principles of laparoscopic procedures, and providing access to the laboratory for familiarization with procedures and their technical considerations. It is usually too late to begin the teaching process when an advanced procedure is about to begin; the whole surgical scenario should have been rehearsed earlier.

N. Katkhouda, *Advanced Laparoscopic Surgery*,
DOI: 10.1007/978-3-540-74843-4_1, © Springer-Verlag Berlin Heidelberg 2011

After completion of basic training in laparoscopic surgery, it is beneficial for nursing staff to attend focused courses. In educational terms, courses intended for nurses and those offered for surgeons can be equally useful.

Following training, it is important to have checklists in the operating room, preferably fixed to the TV monitor, to which nursing staff can refer before and during preparation of the patient. Members of the nursing team should work in harmony, providing understanding and support for each other. The circulating nurse should never leave the operating room without the knowledge and approval of the scrub technician, or more importantly, the surgeon. The surgeon is dependent on the environment, and should an operative problem occur in the absence of the circulating nurse, the smooth rhythm of the operation is threatened.

More than one nursing team should receive appropriate training so that a back up team is always available.

The surgical assistants should also have appropriate training and the above remarks apply equally to this group. They should clearly understand the different steps of the procedure to facilitate a flawless operative process. They should also be taught about potential incidents and complications and be briefed as to what course of action to take.

An advanced surgical procedure will proceed smoothly only if the surgical environment is right. It is the surgeon's responsibility, as team leader, to ensure that all team members have been adequately trained and prepared.

The Instruments

The instruments, the camera, and the video imaging system should all be checked prior to beginning an operation, to ensure that all wiring is connected correctly and all instruments are ready for use. This should be completed preferably half an hour prior to bringing the patient back to the operating room.

Surgeons involved in laparoscopy will each have their preferred list of instruments. This may vary from the standard laparoscopic set which comes in basic and advanced versions:

- The minimum basic set usually consists of trocars, a Veress needle, one right-angle hook, one spatula, one 5 mm dissector, one electrical scissors, one 10 mm Babcock clamp, one cholangiogram clamp, two atraumatic 5 mm graspers, one right-angle dissector, one ratchet grasper, one clip applier, and 0 and 30° 5 or 10 mm laparoscopes.
- The advanced set should include more trocars, two needle holders, two 10 mm Babcock clamps, one 10 mm right-angle dissector, microscissors, sharp scissors, two or three atraumatic graspers, clip appliers (medium and large), laparotie absorbable clips, one needle nose grasper, and harmonic shears.

The basic and advanced trays can naturally be tailored to suit the team's preference, but sets should be standardized to avoid confusion and to make instrument selection and preparation as cost effective as possible. Other specific items needed for a particular procedure should be considered in advance, such as a bag for retrieval of large organs like the spleen. Zero- and 30° 5 and 10 mm laparoscopes should always be available, and an extra camera should be kept in the operating room in case of a technical problem with the original.

There are two basic types of setup, one for upper abdominal surgery and another for lower abdominal surgery.

Setup for Upper Abdominal Surgery

There are two options for laparoscopic cholecystectomy, with modifications for the various advanced laparoscopic procedures.

■ **Basic Laparoscopic Cholecystectomy.** For laparoscopic cholecystectomy the patient is placed in a supine position, with a monitor on each side of the patient at the shoulders.

- The "American" position of the patient. The surgeon stands on the left side of the patient facing a monitor, with the camera assistant to the left of the surgeon. The first assistant is opposite the surgeon on the right side of the patient. The scrub technician will be standing to the right of the first assistant, opposite the surgeon, allowing him or her to hand across instruments appropriately (Fig. 1.1a).
- The "French" position of the patient. The patient can alternatively be positioned with legs spread, the surgeon standing between the legs (inverted Y position). The monitors are on each side of the head of the patient, the camera assistant at the surgeon's right, and the first assistant at the left (Fig. 1.1b). The scrub technician stands at the right side of the surgeon next to the camera assistant. A Mayo stand can be used to position the preferred instruments on the surgeon's right side, where they are easily accessible.

The surgeon should also be able to see vital parameters such as blood pressure, pulse rate, cardiac, and end tidal CO_2 monitoring.

The room therefore should be sufficiently large to allow a virtual division into three sections: one for the anesthesiologist and his or her instrumentation, one for the patient and TV monitors, and the third section for the instrumentation of the scrub technician.

■ **Setup for Advanced Upper Abdominal Surgery.** For all upper gastrointestinal operations the surgeon ideally stands between the patient's legs, facing a TV monitor, with the first assistant to the right and the camera assistant to the left of the patient (Fig. 1.2). This enables the surgeon to have a straight view of the relevant TV monitor. A Mayo stand for the surgeon's instruments is usually placed to the surgeon's right. The scrub technician stands to the left.

For laparoscopic splenectomy the patient is positioned at 60°, using a bean-bag to elevate the left side, with the surgeon standing on the right side of the patient facing a left upper monitor. The first assistant is opposite the surgeon on the patient's left. The camera assistant ideally stands to the left of the surgeon, in which case the scrub technician stands next to the first assistant. The positions are discussed in more detail in the chapter on splenectomy.

It is very important when installing a patient for an advanced upper abdominal procedure to avoid deep venous thrombosis. The patient's legs are spread, the *thighs extended* to avoid a conflict between the knees of the patient and the hands of the surgeon, and the ankles comfortably padded with the use of leg squeezers.

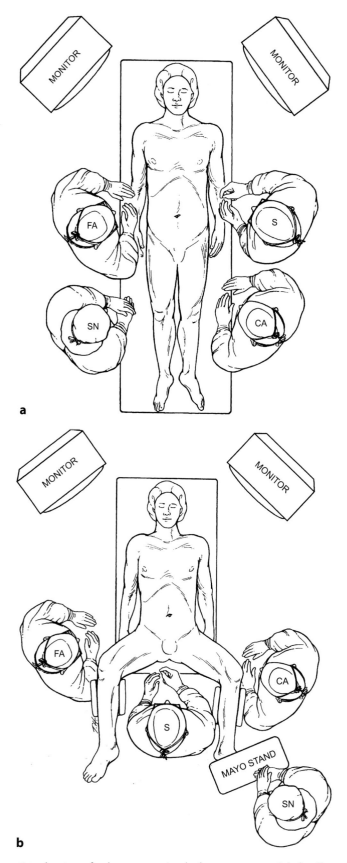

Fig. 1.1 Conventional setups for laparoscopic cholecystectomy: (**a**) the "American" position, and (**b**) the "French" position. *S* surgeon; *FA* first assistant; *SN* scrub nurse; *CA* camera assistant

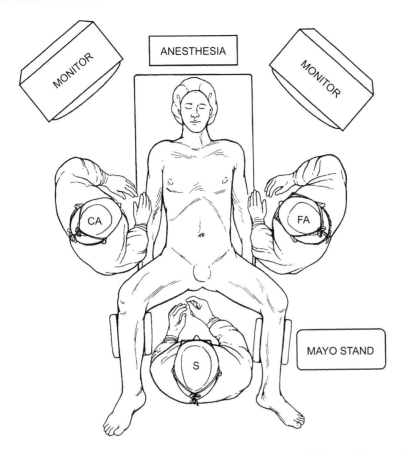

Fig. 1.2 Conventional setup for upper GI surgery. *S* surgeon; *FA* first assistant; *CA* camera assistant

Setup for Lower Abdominal Surgery

For noncolorectal procedures the patient can be placed in a supine position without spreading the legs. In colorectal procedures the patient is placed in a modified Lloyd Davies position with the legs spread. An important aspect here is to make sure that the surgeon can circulate freely, and is able to move from one side of the patient to the other without obstruction from the instrumentation table, or electrocautery, or suction devices.

The monitor is positioned at the feet of the patient for hernia procedures (Fig. 1.3), but for a laparoscopic appendectomy the monitor is placed at the right side of the patient with the surgeon facing the TV monitor (Fig. 1.4). For left sided colorectal procedures, an additional monitor is placed at the patient's left shoulder to allow surgeon visualization when the splenic flexure of the colon is mobilized (Fig. 1.5). The same applies for the right colon and its hepatic flexure, where the monitor should be near the patient's right shoulder (Fig. 1.4).

For laparoscopic hernia repair, it is advised to tuck in both the patient's arms and prepare the patient so the surgeon can alternatively stand on the left or the right.

For laparoscopic appendectomy, the left arm of the patient should be tucked in to allow the surgeon and assistant to stand comfortably on the left side.

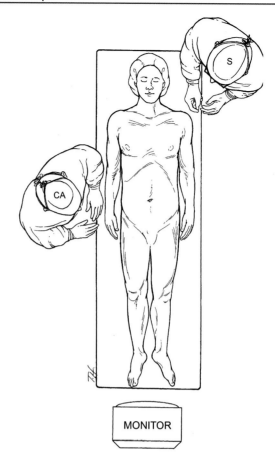

Fig. 1.3 Conventional setup for a hernia repair. *S* surgeon; *CA* camera assistant

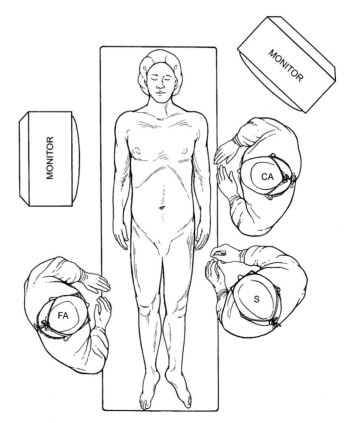

Fig. 1.4 Conventional setup for appendectomy and work on the right colon. *S* surgeon; *FA* first assistant; *CA* camera assistant

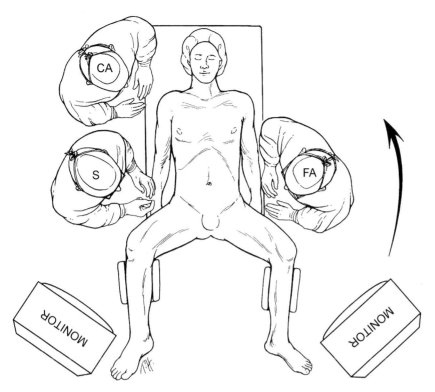

Fig. 1.5 Conventional setup for left colectomy and low anterior resection. *S* surgeon; *FA* first assistant; *CA* camera assistant. *Arrow* indicates movement of monitor

Laparoscopy is performed in a closed abdominal cavity where space is limited. Tilting the operating table so that gravity provides natural retraction by pulling the intraabdominal organs to the lower side can increase available space significantly. It should be possible to position the patient in Trendelenburg or reverse Trendelenburg with either the right side or left side up depending on the procedure, and it is therefore important to use an appropriate table to allow such maneuvers. Some old tables are obsolete and it is worthwhile investing in a modern electrical operative table if one is to embrace advanced laparoscopic surgery.

Laparoscopic surgery demands great concentration. It is therefore important for the operating room to be *quiet* when the surgeon is performing laparoscopic surgery, especially in advanced cases involving knot tying.

The abdomen is a closed unit and the *working space* is a virtual one that has to be created and maintained (Fig. 1.6a–c). The working space can be increased by means of various maneuvers such as tilting the patient – head up or head down, right side up or left side down – where gravity is used to displace adjacent organs from the operating site.

In upper abdominal operations the working space is created by positioning the patient head up to allow the stomach, the colon, and the omental fat to drop down. For hernia repair the patient is placed in a steep Trendelenburg position, so that the small bowel is similarly moved up to free the pelvic area. For colon surgery and appendectomies working space can be created in the same manner, with the addition of lateral tilting of the table to move the

The Working Environment

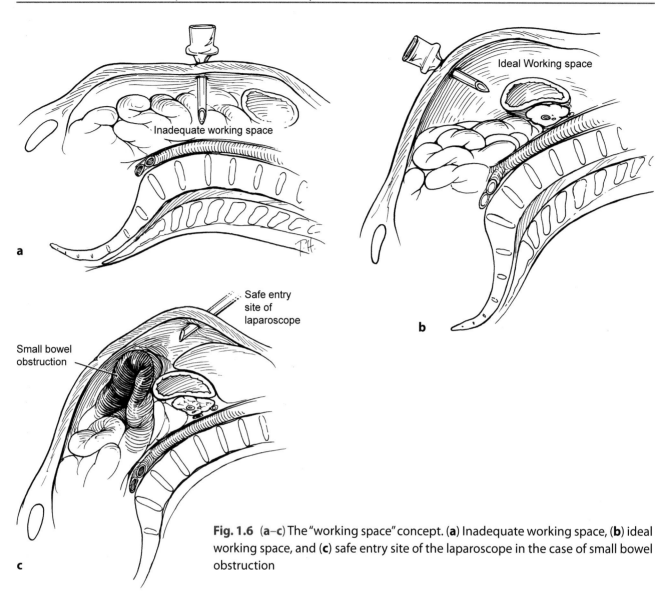

Fig. 1.6 (**a–c**) The "working space" concept. (**a**) Inadequate working space, (**b**) ideal working space, and (**c**) safe entry site of the laparoscope in the case of small bowel obstruction

small bowel away from the operative site. The splenectomy technique also involves creation of working space, with the patient being positioned head up, left side up allowing the stomach and the colon to fall to the right side, giving access to the left hypochondrium.

During a laparoscopic procedure for small bowel obstruction, the same effect can be achieved by tilting the patient to the side opposite the presumed site of the obstruction as indicated by the preoperative physical examination and abdominal plain films.

The working space concept is especially important upon inserting the laparoscope. If the working space is severely limited, as, for example, with small bowel obstruction, it is easy to injure the bowel with placement of the first trocar. For this reason, flexibility in the choice of trocar insertion sites is recommended, following the simple principle of triangulation that governs all trocar insertions.

If the maximum pressure of 15 mmHg is reached with a flow of less than 2 L of CO_2 upon insertion of the first trocar, one should convert to an open procedure as this indicates that there will not be adequate working space due to the distended bowel.

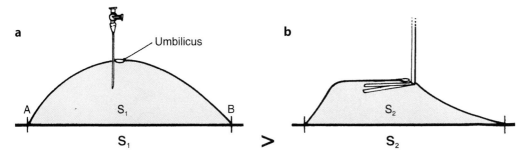

Fig. 1.7 Comparison of (**a**) pneumoperitoneum, created with a Varess needle, and (**b**) gasless laparoscopy. *S* surface

Appraisal of Surgical Instruments

The working space concept also explains difficulties of working in a gasless environment where the shape of the abdomen, once retracted with a gasless device, is not round but more trapezoidal (Fig. 1.7). This does not provide adequate working space, and is one of the reasons for which gasless laparoscopy has been abandoned.

Trocars

■ **Choosing an Appropriate Trocar.** There is no ideal trocar size. Ten-millimeter trocars are recommended for most advanced procedures as they allow flexibility and use of different diameters of scissors, clip appliers, and other instruments. Advanced surgeons can also use 5 mm trocars for advanced cases to improve cosmesis but the 5 mm instruments tend to be less blunt and possibly more traumatic than larger 10 mm instruments when used to dissect planes.

The 5 mm trocars are routinely used for basic laparoscopic cholecystectomies, laparoscopic hernia procedures, and laparoscopic appendectomies. These smaller trocars leave barely visible marks and are ideal as supplemental trocars whenever needed in any advanced procedure.

There has been a recent trend towards the use of smaller trocars, even for advanced procedures. Microlaparoscopy has also been offered as an option in selected cases using 2–3 mm trocars.

There is some discussion over the issue of disposable vs. nondisposable trocars, but the author's preference is for the disposable variety. These have safety shields, and if they are manipulated appropriately they will serve their purpose and intraabdominal injuries can be avoided.

■ **Disposable Trocars.** The critical maneuver when inserting disposable trocars is to retract the abdominal wall manually, to increase the distance between the abdominal wall and the intraabdominal organs, and to create a virtual space that is otherwise absent. If this is not done, the trocar will push the abdominal wall during insertion and may injure intraabdominal organs and even major vessels such as the aorta (Fig. 1.8). Disposable trocars should be held firmly in the palm and not in a pencil fashion as advised by some companies. Most of the force should come from the shoulder and not the forearm.

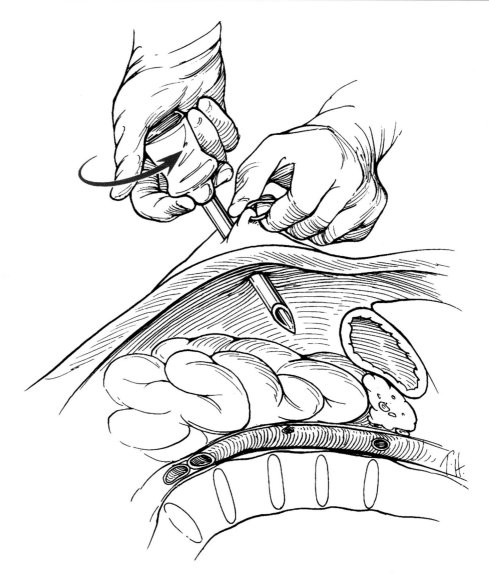

Fig. 1.8 Creation of working space in the abdomen

A conical blade shape is a better choice than a pyramidal shape because it pushes the tissue upon insertion and avoids laceration. The general movement of insertion is a slight clockwise screwing motion with very little pushing of the right hand, and fixation by the left hand, as shown in Fig. 1.8.

■ **Nondisposable Trocars.** These are now rarely used in the United States due to concerns over blood-borne pathogens, although they are still in use in European and other countries. To avoid herniation, a "Z" entry of the fascial layers was promoted by Kurt Semm (Fig. 1.9).

■ **Optical Viewing Trocars.** The optiview trocars have the advantage of allowing entry into the abdomen under direct laparoscopic guidance. In theory this should avoid the injury of superficial vessels crossing the fascia, and provide awareness of penetration of the peritoneal cavity. This is a useful advantage. The author's preference goes to these types of trocars, as they enhance safety during their insertion.

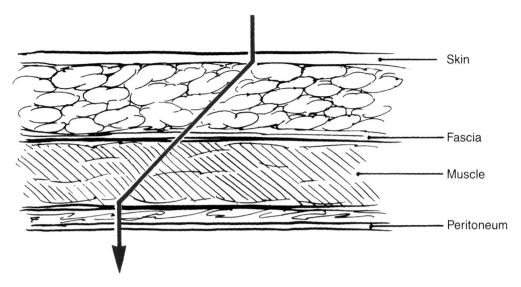

Fig. 1.9 "Z" entry of the fascial layers with a nondisposable trocar

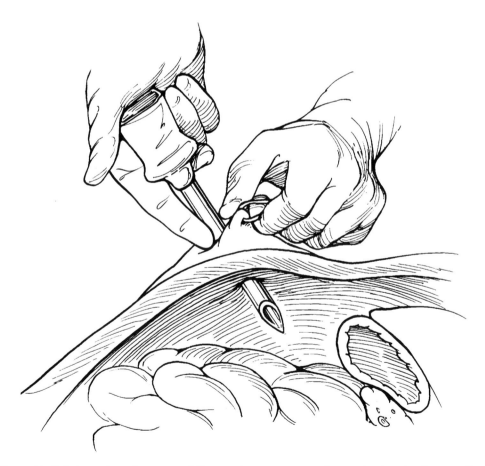

Fig. 1.10 Safe insertion of a trocar while exerting countertraction and using the *finger* to limit the thrust

■ **Prevention of Accidents with Trocars.** It cannot be overemphasized that caution is essential to avoid injuries when using any kind of trocar. The surgeon should be very cautious not to insert the full length of the trocar, and always to keep at least half of the shaft outside the abdomen until a laparoscope is inserted and the intraperitoneal space is visualized. It is safer to have a trocar stuck midway in the fascia than midway in an abdominal organ. After palming the trocar, a finger is placed above the tip to act as an additional safety measure (Fig. 1.10). A useful tip is to insert the video laparoscope in the trocar if the localization of the trocar and the intraabdominal situation is not clear. One can then check whether the trocar is still in the fascia and muscles. This works on a principle similar to the optical viewing trocar.

■ **Triangulation of Trocars.** It is also noted that the trocars are not only inserted at a 90° angle to the camera, but may also point in a triangular fashion towards the target inside the abdomen (Fig. 1.11 dotted lines) (*double triangulation*).

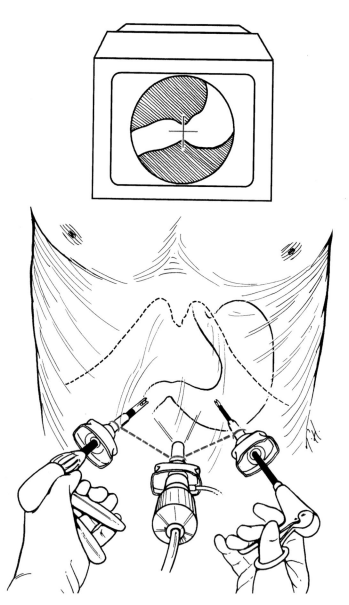

Fig. 1.11 Double "triangulation" during trocar insertion

Other Instrumental Requirements

■ **Laparoscopes.** It is often said that the 30° laparoscope should be reserved for use by the "professional" laparoscopic surgeon, while the 0° laparoscope is the best choice for the "amateur" laparoscopic surgeon. This is not always true! There are some major differences between the two types which dictate their ideal usage:

- The 0° laparoscope has a bright picture with a large panoramic view. Its vertical lens has less contact with intraabdominal organs and therefore does not dirty as quickly.
- In contrast, the 30° instrument has a less bright picture and more limited image width. It also has the disadvantage of getting dirty more often, especially in an obese patient, because of the special angle of the lens which often rubs on the intraabdominal fat. Its use also requires more skill from the camera operator.

On the other hand, a major advantage of the 30° scope is that it allows the visualization of structures and vision of angles that are not possible with a 0° laparoscope, and this is especially true for advanced laparoscopic procedures.

It is recommended that both types of cameras be available, allowing the surgeon to begin with the 0° one and switch to the 30°. The 30° laparoscope is also recommended for surgery on organs that have special requirements, such as laparoscopic splenectomy, especially for control of the hilar vessels.

As a rule of thumb, a 30° scope is probably more useful than a 0° type. We have also used a 45° laparoscope during obesity surgery when a critical view of the gastrojejunostomy is required. All laparoscopes should be kept warm ready for use, and for this purpose a *special Thermos bottle* is a very useful investment. The habit of using a "Fred" device to defog a laparoscope is not based on any scientific data. It is known that the single most important factor to avoid fogging is to keep the temperature of the laparoscope the same as the intraabdominal temperature. This is best done by leaving the unused laparoscope in a Thermos bottle with very warm water. It is also advisable to start the case with a warm laparoscope to avoid fogging and hence time wasted in defogging.

It is also advisable to make sure that the room temperature is adequate, especially when performing long advanced laparoscopic procedures. There will be a tendency for the laparoscope to cool down and fog every time it is cleaned or taken out of the abdomen. This should be explained to the scrub technician, the circulating nurse, and the camera assistant.

Laparoscopes should be checked frequently to ensure they are in proper working order. Lenses should not be cleaned with rough materials, such as standard surgical gauze. Appropriate smooth gauze should be used and will protect the laparoscope and gentle handling is necessary so as not to bend the telescope. A breakdown of the lenses inside the laparoscope will hinder vision and detract from the quality of the video recording.

■ **Cameras.** Two parameters dictate the quality of a camera:

- Definition and contrast
- Natural color discrimination and reproduction

It is very difficult to give advice on the most appropriate camera, but it is the author's opinion that standard "single-chip" cameras are not suitable for advanced laparoscopic surgery. The definition and color analysis is not sufficient for delicate structures.

"Three-chip" cameras have better color definition but they are currently more expensive and are heavier. A lightweight three-chip (3CCD) *high-definition* 1080p camera is ideal (Karl Storz, Tuttlingen, Germany). Light-carrying cables should be checked regularly to ensure that all the fiber optics contained in the cable are still functioning and not broken, otherwise the amount of light brought to the camera will not be sufficient and vision will be hindered. This is the most common problem with light cords.

Creation of the Pneumo-peritoneum

There are two basic techniques for creating pneumoperitoneum. One is an open surgical technique using a Hasson trocar; the other is a closed technique using a Veress needle. Each method has advantages and disadvantages. The author personally uses the closed technique with a Veress needle, and in more than 20 years of advanced laparoscopy performing several thousand procedures, the author has experienced only one injury (on a distended stomach on his third laparoscopic case in 1989).

When a Veress needle is used, the author recommends that a nasogastric tube be inserted into the stomach and the stomach deflated so as to avoid puncture. When performing lower abdominal surgery it is also important to insert a urinary catheter. A small incision is made in the umbilicus. The skin around the incision is grasped with one hand and lifted up, and the Veress needle is then slowly inserted. Care is needed to make sure that the red line of the Veress needle (when using a disposable version) appears during fascial penetration; a sudden disappearance of the red line is accompanied by a noise that will indicate that the needle is in the abdomen. If the needle is *not* in the virtual abdominal space but is in a fatty intraabdominal deposit, the red line will move up and down indicating incorrect placement of the needle. In all cases a confirmatory test should be performed using saline or preferably an empty syringe. An empty 10 cm³ syringe fixed on the needle is first aspirated to make sure that there is no intraabdominal fluid coming from the needle – such as blood, bowel content, or bile. Ten cubic centimeter of air is then injected into the peritoneal cavity; if it cannot be aspirated back the injected air must have diffused into the cavity and the needle is properly placed. If the injected air comes back into the syringe the needle is not in the peritoneal cavity, and so it should be pushed a little further.

It is imperative *not* to insert the full length of the needle, and to perform the syringe test before hooking up the tubing of the CO_2 tank. When the needle is correctly placed, the CO_2 tubing is attached to the needle and insufflation can begin. A low gas flow (or no flow) with high pressure indicates that the needle is not in the abdomen. At this point the

CO_2 should be discontinued and the position of the needle should be checked again. It is advisable to change the position of the needle using the same skin incision but in another direction. It is also possible to change from the umbilical site to the left upper quadrant (Palmer's point). After three failed attempts, the general rule is that one should convert to an open laparoscopy procedure using a Hasson trocar.

An open laparoscopy technique requires a small fascial incision. The two edges are then grasped and sutures placed in the fascia. The Hassan open trocar is inserted under direct vision and the ties secured to the trocar.

Direct closed laparoscopy with the insertion of a trocar *without* pneumoperitoneum (not to be confused with gasless laparoscopy where no trocars are used at all), as advocated by some gynecologists, is dangerous and should never be used under any circumstances.

Troubleshooting Loss of Pneumoperitoneum

Occasionally during a laparoscopic case, the surgeon may feel that there is no working space. Usually this is secondary to loss of pneumoperitoneum. The knowledge and interpretation of the indicators on the insufflation unit will determine the origin of the problem and how to address it. Here are explanations of several common scenarios:

1. Pressure higher than 15 mmHg
(a) Patient is not fully paralyzed or is waking up during the surgery
(b) Pressure is set higher than 15 mmHg
(c) The trocar valve is closed or there is a kink in the tube
2. Pressure is lower than 15
(a) The flow is 0
    i.   Gas tank is empty
(b) The flow is high
    i.   The tube is disconnected
    ii. One of the trocar valves is open
    iii. The suction is working and is stronger than the insufflator

Control of Bleeding of Unnamed Vessels

An unnamed vessel can be controlled in the same manner as a main vessel (see below), but usually simple compression with an atraumatic clamp and careful electrocautery will control the bleeding, so long as the major abdominal organs are kept under vision at an appropriate distance.

Compression is one of the best possible means of achieving hemostasis on a rough surface. One should use a 2×2 in. laparoscopic gauze that is radiopaque and also contains a thread that will enable it to be visualized laparoscopically (e.g., Wecksorb 2×2 gauze by Pilling Weck, Inc.) (Fig. 1.12a). This compression follows the principles of open surgery, namely temporary hemostasis allowing cleaning of the area and identification of the nature of the bleeding.

Principles of Hemostasis

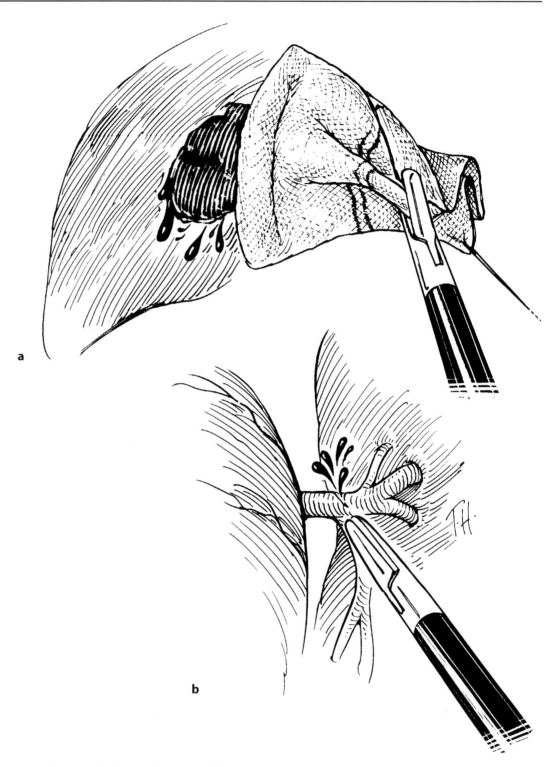

a

b

Fig. 1.12 (**a**, **b**) Techniques of hemostasis: (**a**) compression with 2×2 gauze; (**b**) forceps control

Compression is achieved by the surgeon's left hand, leaving the right hand free to insert the irrigation suction device, aspirate the blood, and make sure that the area is clean while the compression is maintained and a decision is made as to what tool will be used to ensure hemostasis, Usually a flat spatula will control the problem; but if it is to be used on an organ such as the liver or the spleen, high-voltage monopolar electrical current should be applied with caution, avoiding adjacent organs. It is critical to keep the bleeding space dry while applying the electrical surgical current by suctioning constantly as the electrical current is applied.

Control of Bleeding of a Main Named Vessel

There is a major difference between handling a hemorrhage from a main vessel and that from an unnamed vessel. A main vessel requires vascular compression, retraction of the camera to protect the lens from splashing blood, and irrigation of the field. An attempt then be made to secure the hemostasis with clips. The surgeon should never attempt to clip a main vessel blindly in a bloody operating site, as visceral injuries will occur.

For bleeding originating from a main abdominal vessel, compression *cannot* be applied using 2×2 gauze. Instead it is necessary to use a large atraumatic clamp such as a small-bowel clamp or long Kelly with atraumatic jaws and tips that will compress the bleeding structure and its surrounding structures (Fig. 1.12b). Gentle and atraumatic application will avoid injuring or rupturing the vessel itself. The same procedure as above is then followed: cleaning, aspiration, irrigation, and application of clips, electrical current, or a suture, depending on the situation.

A vessel should not be divided before its proximal and distal ends are identified and the vessel has been controlled without incorporating adjacent structures in the clips.

Electrocautery can be performed using either monopolar or bipolar current. The use of monopolar current carries the risk of intraabdominal diffusion and transmission of power to adjacent structures. During application of monopolar current other organs should not be touched and the tip of the electrocautery instrument should be kept under direct vision at all times. This is especially true when using monopolar current in conjunction with scissors with long blades or long noninsulated instruments. The risk of intraabdominal explosion is more theoretical than real and has not occurred in the author's practice, but the use of nitrous oxide in this setting is not recommended because it supports combustion.

Bipolar instruments are probably safer but have the disadvantage of producing more smoke and are slower to achieve hemostasis. Of the available bipolar instruments, bipolar scissors and bipolar grasping forceps are the most useful and should be available in advanced laparoscopic trays.

Harmonic shears (also known as harmonic scalpel, Ethicon EndoSurgery, Inc.) with vibrating blades oscillate at 50,000 cycles a second, producing heat by friction and resulting in a coagulation process that can seal structures such as small ducts or small vessels. Harmonic shears can also be used on most of the unnamed vessels, up to a diameter of 5 mm, above which it is safer to apply clips or ties.

Irrigation and Suction Devices

Many irrigation/suction devices are available. Ideally such a device should deliver appropriate irrigation at *variable* flow rates, with the possibility of hydrodissection if required.

The suction component of irrigation systems is its Achilles heel because the suction pipe is usually connected to the central facility on the operating room wall. Suction is therefore too strong and will simply suck away the pneumoperitoneum, immediately obscuring the view before achieving a result. As a result the suction force has to be made adjustable, usually using small forceps, especially when suction is immediately needed (as for hemorrhage).

The tip of the suction cannula is usually sharp and can traumatize tissues or vessels. The handpiece containing the valve has to be small, and is held ergonomically in the palm of the hand with separate trumpets for suction and irrigation.

Finally, many devices offer the possibility of insertion of standard laparoscopic instruments through a large (10 mm) shaft but the complexity of the mounting has prevented its generalized adoption.

Ammori BJ, Morais JC (1996) A simple method of closure of a laparoscopic trocar site. J R Coll Surg Edinb 41(2):120–121

Berguer R, Rab GT, Abu-Ghaida H, Alarcon A, Chung J (1987) A comparison of surgeons' posture during laparoscopic and open surgical procedures. Surg Endosc 11(2):139–142

Castellvi AO, Hollett LA, Minhajuddin A, Hogg DC, Tesfay ST, Scott DJ (2009) Maintaining proficiency after fundamentals of laparoscopic surgery training: a 1-year analysis of skill retention for surgery residents. Surgery 146(2):387–393

Chaloner EJ, Heath AD (1996) Technique for closure of port sites under laparoscopic visual control [comment]. Br J Surg 83(1):134–135

Champion JK, Hunter J, Trus T, Laycock W (1996) Teaching basic video skills as an aid in laparoscopic suturing. Surg Endosc 10(1):23–25

Chung RS (1995) Closure of trocar wounds in laparoscopic operations. The threading technique. Surg Endosc 9(5):534–536

Conlon KC, Curtin I (1995) A simple technique for the closure of laparoscopic trocar wounds. J Am Coll Surg 181(6):565–566

Curtis P, Bournas N, Magos A (1995) Simple equipment to facilitate operative laparoscopic surgery (or how to avoid a spaghetti junction). Br J Obstet Gynaecol 102(6):495–497

DesCoteaux JG, Tye L, Poulin EC (1996) Reuse of disposable laparoscopic instruments: cost analysis. Can J Surg 39(2):133–139

Elashry OM, Nakada SY, Wolf JS Jr, Figenshau RS, McDougall EM, Clayman RV (1996) Comparative clinical study of port-closure techniques following laparoscopic surgery. J Am Coll Surg 183(4):335–344

Feldman LS, Cao J, Andalib A, Fraser S, Fried GM (2009) A method to characterize the learning curve for performance of a fundamental laparoscopic simulator task: defining "learning plateau" and "learning rate". Surgery 146(2):381–386

Frangov T, Mladenov V, Mouiel J, Katkhouda N (1994) Diagnostic laparoscopy and laparoscopic surgery, their development and outlook. Khirurgiia 47:(1):28–30 (in Bulgarian)

Fried GM, Clas D, Meakins JL (1994) Minimally invasive surgery in the elderly patient. Surg Clin North Am 74(2):375–387

Hirvonen EA, Nuutinen LS, Kauko M (1995) Hemodynamic changes due to Trendeienburg positioning and pneumoperitoneum during laparoscopic hysterectomy. Acta Anaesthesiol Scand 39(7):949–955

James AW, Rabl C, Westphalen AC, Fogarty PF, Posselt AM, Campos GM (2009) Portomesenteric venous thrombosis after laparoscopic surgery: a systematic literature review. Arch Surg 144(6):520–526

Katkhouda N, Lord RV (2000) Once more with feeling. Handoscopy or the rediscovery of the virtues of the surgeon's hands. Surg Endosc 14:985–986

Kavoussi LR, Moore RG, Adams JB, Partin AW (1995) Comparison of robotic versus human laparoscopic camera control. J Urol 154(6):2134–2136

Korndorffer JR Jr, Scott DJ, Sierra R, Brunner WC, Dunne JB, Slakey DP, Townsend MC, Hewitt RL (2005) Developing and testing competency levels for laparoscopic skills training. Arch Surg 140(1):80–84

Meyers W, Katkhouda N (1999) Handoscopic surgery: a prospective multi-center trial of a minimally invasive technique for complex abdominal surgery. Southern Surgeon's Club Study Group. Arch Surg 134:477–483

Robertson GS, Lloyd DM, Kelly MJ, Veitch PS (1996) Technique for full-thickness muscle closure of laparoscopic port sites. Br J Surg 83(3):383

Rosser JC, Rosser LE, Savalgi RS (1997) Skill acquisition and assessment for laparoscopic surgery. Arch Surg 132(2):200–204

Schaer GN, Koechli OR, Hailer U (1995) Single-use versus reusable laparoscopic surgical instruments: a comparative cost analysis. Am J Obstet Gynecol 173(6):1812–1815

Stebbing JF, Mortensen NJ (1995) Use of video-laparoscope to shed light on conventional pelvic dissection. Br J Surg 82(7):902

Stefanidis D, Heniford BT (2009) The formula for a successful laparoscopic skills curriculum. Arch Surg 144(1):77–82

Stringer NH, Levy ES, Kezmoh MP, Walker J, Abramovitz S, Sadowski DL, Kefiemariam Y (1995) New closure technique for lateral operative laparoscopic trocar sites. A report of 80 closures. Surg Endosc 9(7):838–840

Targarona EM, Gracia E, Rodriguez M, Cerdán G, Balagué C, Garriga J, Trias M (2003) Hand-assisted laparoscopic surgery. Arch Surg 138(2):133–141

Udwadia TE, Udwadia RT (1994) Patient position for laparoscopic surgery. Surg Endosc 8(9):1129–1130

Unger S, Olsen D, Nagy A, Zucker K, Katkhouda N (1994) Laparoscopic surgery: surgical education, The People Republic of China. Surg Laparosc Endosc 4:277–283

Weber DM (2003) Laparoscopic surgery: an excellent approach in elderly patients. Arch Surg 138(10):1083–1088

Zucker KA, Bailey RW, Graham SM et al (1993) Training for laparoscopic surgery. World J Surg 17:3–7

Cholecystectomy 2

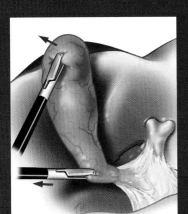

The patient is placed in the supine position with either the left arm or both arms tucked. The surgeon stands on the left and the assistant stands on the right side of the patient. The camera assistant stands on the left side of the patient to the left of the surgeon, or alternatively the assistant may hold the camera from the other side of the table (on the right side of the patient) if there is no dedicated camera assistant.

The abdomen can be entered using the Hasson technique or the Veress needle. After insertion of the umbilical trocar for the laparoscope, the remaining trocars should be introduced taking into account the patient's body habitus. A standardized routine may be used for trocar insertion, but should be adapted based on patient size. For example if patient is obese, the trocars should be placed closer to the costal margin (Fig. 2.1).

After the abdomen is insufflated, the patient is positioned in reverse Trendelenburg and right side up. This ensures that the duodenum and transverse colon are moved down by gravity and improves exposure. The next trocar to be inserted is the lateral trocar used to retract the fundus and inspect the triangle of Calot. Adhesions in this region may influence subsequent trocar position. Quite often this trocar is inserted too low so that the grasper cannot reach the liver, and thus is unable to flip the gallbladder together with the liver to ensure proper exposure. For this reason it is recommended that the first 5 mm trocar be inserted just under the right costal margin and as laterally as possible. Before insertion it is also necessary to ensure that the handle of the grasper is not blocked by the patient's flank or knees. Pushing the abdominal wall with the left hand will indent the abdomen and help ideal placement of the trocars by visualization of the entry site.

The next trocar to be inserted is a 10–12 mm trocar and forms the operating port. It is usually inserted to the right of the falciform ligament, just at the level of the border of the right lobe of the liver. If the trocar is inserted more laterally there is a risk of injury

Basic Laparoscopic Cholecystectomy

N. Katkhouda, *Advanced Laparoscopic Surgery*,
DOI: 10.1007/978-3-540-74843-4_2, © Springer-Verlag Berlin Heidelberg 2011

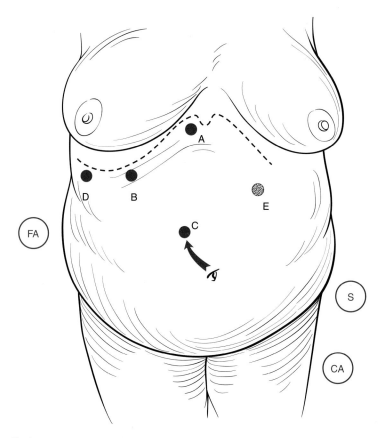

Fig. 2.1 Cholecystectomy in the obese patient; *arrow* indicates camera port moved higher and to the right, toward the right costal margin. *A* subxyphoid trocar for instrument; *B* midclavicular port for left hand of surgeon; *D* grasper for retraction of gallbladder; *E* additional standard port for obese. *S* surgeon; *FA* first assistant; *CA* camera assistant

to the superior epigastric vessels, which can lead to severe hemorrhage. If this trocar is too low, however, the angle of dissection will be incorrect and there will be conflict with the laparoscope ("knitting needle" effect).

Once the operating port has been inserted, the fundus of the gallbladder is retracted and an additional 5 mm trocar is inserted for lateral retraction of Hartmann's pouch. The operating port, the video laparoscope, and the lateral trocar are triangulated to avoid a "knitting needle" effect between the graspers and the video laparoscope (Fig. 2.2a).

In the case of an obese patient, the surgeon should not struggle to try to retract the fat. Two tricks can be used:

- Placing the patient on steep reverse Trendelenburg
- Inserting an extra 5 mm trocar above and to the left of the umbilical trocar (Fig. 2.1)

This additional trocar can be very helpful. If used, it should be added at an early stage, permitting the insertion of an irrigation/suction device, which can be used as a retractor to push down the duodenum and the greater omentum. It will also serve for hydrodissection. This extra trocar should be used for all obese patients, and also when the duodenum is stuck to the gallbladder and the surgeon requires extra duodenal retraction. The

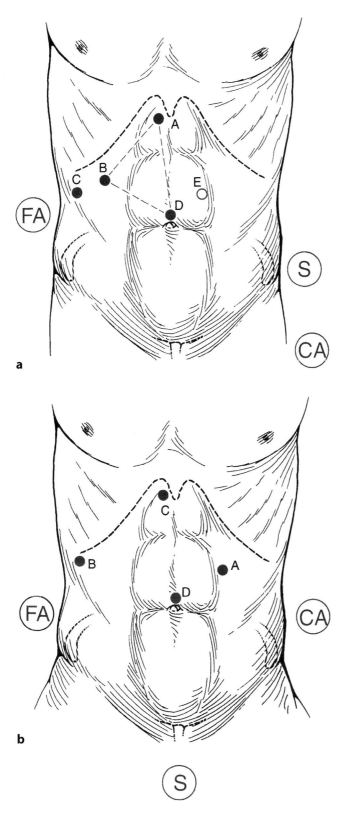

Fig. 2.2 Ideal port placement for laparoscopic cholecystectomy. (**a**) The "American" trocar placement, the surgeon standing at the side, and (**b**) the "French" trocar placement, the surgeon standing between the legs of the patient. *A* operating port; *B* grasper for the surgeon; *C* grasper/ liver retractor; *D* umbilical telescope; *E* additional trocar for an obese patient. *S* surgeon; *FA* first assistant; *CA* camera assistant

insertion of the extra 5 mm trocar will not affect the surgical result or the cosmetic appearance but will dramatically increase the safety of the procedure and reduce operative time.

Once the fundus of the gallbladder is retracted and the liver is moved up, some adhesions on the inferior surface of the liver will occasionally prevent adequate liver retraction. Such adhesions should be removed *first* before even attempting dissection of the triangle of Calot, as at this point of the procedure, maximal superior retraction of the gallbladder is needed.

Lateral retraction is the key to safe dissection of the triangle of Calot (Fig. 2.3a). This is performed with the left hand of the surgeon pulling laterally and inferiorly (towards the right Anterior Superior Iliac Spine) on Hartmann's pouch while the first assistant retracts the fundus of the gallbladder towards the lateral right hemidiaphragm. This will open up the triangle of Calot and the risk of a common bile duct (CBD) injury will be minimized. Wrong retraction closing the angle between the cystic duct and the CBD is depicted in Fig. 2.3b. If the anterior peritoneum overlying the cystic duct and artery is scarred, it is very important to retract the cystic duct in a cephalad direction and incise the posterior peritoneum as closely as possible to the neck of the gallbladder. That will allow safe dissection of the cystic duct next to the neck of the gallbladder, and will create a window around the cystic duct.

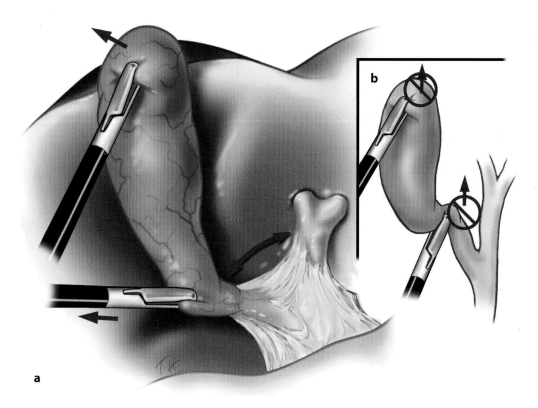

Fig. 2.3 Dissection of the triangle of Calot: (**a**) correct retraction; (**b**) incorrect retraction with the risk of injury to the common bile duct (CBD)

to make a small opening using electrical scissors and insert an irrigation suction device into the fundus to aspirate the contents of the gallbladder. This will ease the tension of the gallbladder and enable it to be grasped using graspers with tiny teeth.

With a very difficult acute gangrenous gallbladder, it is essential for safety reasons to prevent injury to the CBD by limiting dissection to the neck of the gallbladder. The dissection can then proceed as for a normal gallbladder. It is important to visualize the CBD laparoscopically. If this is not possible secondary to inflammation in the porta hepatis, then *a cholangiogram* should be attempted through the neck of the gallbladder to visualize the anatomy. However, if this also is not feasible, and the cystic duct and the neck of the gallbladder have been clearly identified, then one can proceed with the cholecystectomy. It is also possible to perform a cholangiogram through the gallbladder itself. As a rule of thumb the aim should be to recognize the elements of the triangle of Calot within 45 min of beginning the dissection. If after that period of time the anatomy is still not clear, *conversion should be the rule.*

As the gallbladder is being removed from the liver bed some bleeding may occur from the liver parenchyma, owing to difficulty in finding the best plane of dissection. Compression should be applied using a 2 × 2 gauze, and a collagen hemostatic pad should be left in place on the liver bed.

"Dangerous" Cholecystectomy

In some cases of gangrenous gallbladder there may not be an obvious plane of dissection. If the surgeon has limited skills, or feels that the situation is dangerous, he or she should perform a partial removal of the gallbladder, leaving part of its neck next to the CBD.

This is also true when the cystic duct is either atrophic, extremely short, or virtually absent owing to the amount of inflammation. If the cystic duct is very large, one should not apply clips that will not hold; instead, it is preferable to use a preformed Endoloop, create a knot using extracorporeal techniques, or perform intracorporeal suturing using a 3–0 PDS to close the large cystic duct (Fig. 2.7).

Impacted Stone (Hydrops, Empyema, Early Mirizzi)

In the case of a stone impacted in the neck of the gallbladder with an empyema or hydrops of the gallbladder (Fig. 2.8), a good technique is to aspirate the gallbladder after opening the fundus with hot scissors and introducing the irrigation suction canula in the opening. An incision is then made in the neck of the gallbladder, approximately two to three centimeters above the junction of the cystic duct and the neck. This incision should be generous to allow for exteriorization of the stone, almost like an "enucleation" of a mass (Fig. 2.9). Once this is performed, the cystic duct is often shortened or absent. The junction between the neck of the gallbladder and the hepatic duct is also shortened and dangerous for dissection. We recommend in this case completing the opening of the gallbladder, and obtaining a mushroom shape of Hartmann's pouch that will be closed using a running suture after the removal of the rest of the gallbladder (subtotal cholecystectomy), (Fig. 2.10). The placement of a JP drain is also advisable.

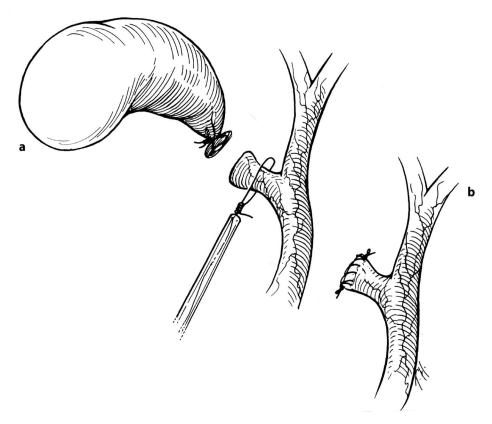

Fig. 2.7 The "dangerous" cholecystectomy: closure of the cystic duct (**a**) using an Endoloop; (**b**) intracorporeal suturing

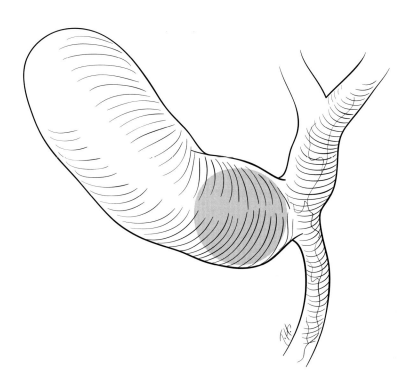

Fig. 2.8 Impacted stone in the neck of the gallbladder (hydrops or empyema)

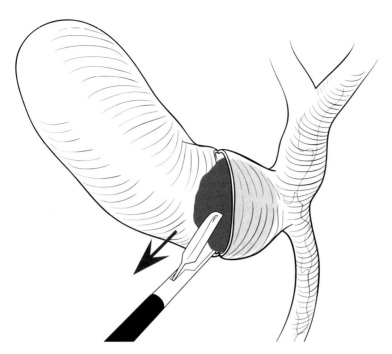

Fig. 2.9 "Enucleation" of impacted stone in the neck of the gallbladder

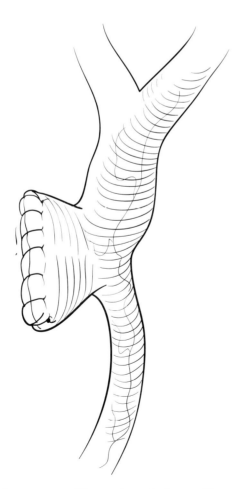

Fig. 2.10 "Subtotal cholecystectomy." Preserving a "safety wall" represented by Hartmann's pouch nearly fused with CBD

Avoiding Injury to the Common Bile Duct

In most instances, an injury to the CBD occurs when the cystic duct is shortened or virtually absent secondary to an anomaly in the anatomy, or in the case of acute inflammation. It is also important to remember that most CBD injuries occur in so-called "simple cholecystectomies" with a minimally inflamed gallbladder. The figures depict the common mechanisms of clipping and injuring the CBD. The fat present at the hepatic duct does not allow for perfect visualization of the cystic duct. In Fig. 2.11a, the fat covers a normal length cystic duct. In Fig. 2.11b, tissue and fat cover a short or absent cystic duct. Both cases present themselves in an identical manner on the screen to the eye of the surgeon who has a two dimensional vision lacking the perception of depth. A clip is placed at what is considered to be the neck of the gallbladder, and an incision is made for a possible cholangiogram. In the first example, the clip is placed across the neck of the gallbladder, and the

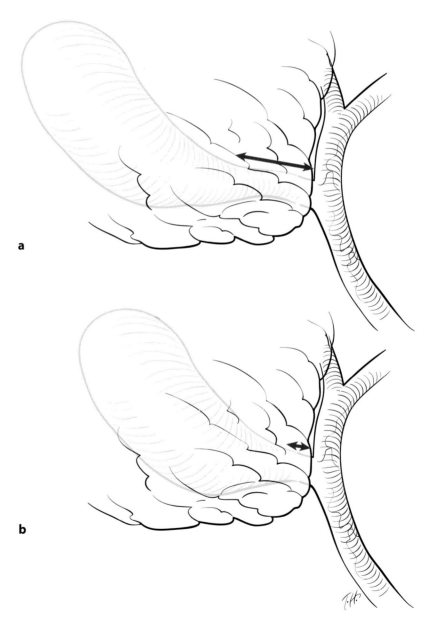

Fig. 2.11 **(a)** Represents a *classic* cystic duct with *normal length*, covered by some tissue and fat. **(b)** Represents a "dangerous" *short* or *absent* duct

incision is made in the cystic duct. In the second example, the cystic duct is shortened and the incision has been made in the CBD, thus injuring the bile duct (Fig. 2.12b). Figures 2.13a, b clearly illustrate through color coding the visual confusion as a consequence of the shortened or absent cystic duct, leading to a CBD injury. In our opinion, these figures indicate the need for a very thorough dissection of the neck of the gallbladder, the junction between the cystic duct and neck of the gallbladder, and the junction between the cystic duct and the hepatic duct (visual cholangiogram). This "double safety" feature (dissection of the junction neck of the gallbladder and cystic duct and dissection of the junction cystic duct, hepatic duct) in addition to the lateral traction will minimize the risk of a CBD injury.

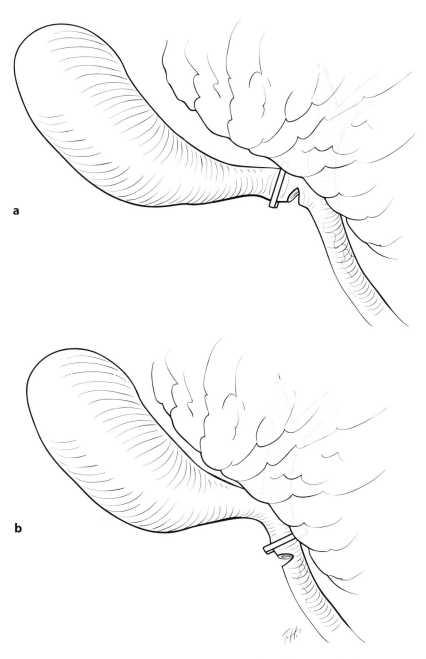

Fig. 2.12 Mechanisms of injury to the CBD. (**a**) Clip placed appropriately across cystic duct. (**b**) Clip placed across the CBD (short or absent cystic duct)

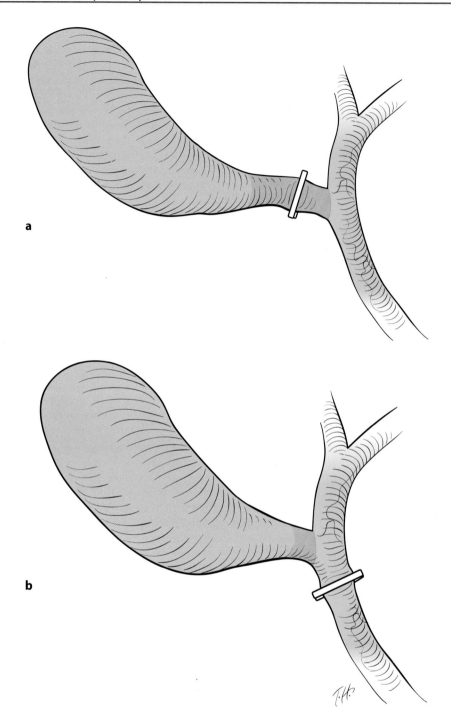

Fig. 2.13 (**a**, **b**) Mechanisms of injury to the CBD. Color coding illustrates the illusion created by the short cystic duct

If hemorrhage occurs from the liver bed, the spatula used to dissect the gallbladder can conveniently be used to attempt hemostasis, with an increase in voltage from the cautery unit. If there is *severe* bleeding in the liver bed, it is possible to introduce a piece of 2 × 2 radiopaque gauze and apply compression. The steps of managing hemorrhage from the liver bed are:

- Avoid obscuring the video laparoscope with blood, pull the camera back, leaving the tip in the port to still provide adequate visualization.
- Compress the bleeding with 2 × 2 gauze if available.
- Irrigate and clean the area around the bleeding.
- Remove the gauze.
- Introduce an irrigation/suction device to dry the site of bleeding with the left hand.
- Apply high-current electrocautery with the spatula using the right hand. This current creates a crust that halts the bleeding. Care is taken to check that the tip of the cautery does not injure a peripheral bile duct (Duct of Lushka). This can be the cause of postoperative bile leak.

Application of clips is usually a waste of time as it is rarely efficient in controlling oozing in the liver bed.

If these actions do not initially take care of the bleeding the compression should be continued. Hemostatic agents such as Tisseal or Floseal (Baxter Inc, Deerfield, IL) can be used to achieve hemostasis.

If the bleeding is due to a major tear in the liver, and hepatic or portal venous branches are involved, and if all possibilities are exhausted, the only recourse is conversion using a mini-laparotomy. This has very rarely been the case in the author's experience, but it may occur more frequently in cirrhotic patients. There is no need for a large subcostal incision and usually a 5 cm mini-laparotomy will suffice.

In the case of a supra-umbilical incision with severe midline adhesions that obscure the view, one can place a 5 mm trocar along the left midclavicular line to take those adhesions down using harmonic shears (Fig. 2.14). Another trick is to insert the camera to the right and superior to the umbilicus, closer to the gallbladder. The patient is tilted to the left, possibly on a bean bag; this will allow for a different angle of visualization and a safe cholecystectomy. Trocars for the right and left hand are also placed a little more to the right of the patient (Fig. 2.15).

Controlling Bleeding in the Liver Bed

Adhesions Due to Previous Upper Midline Laparotomy

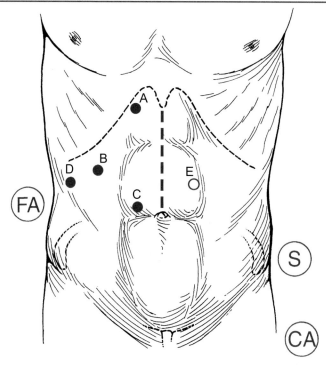

Fig. 2.14 Cholecystectomy in a patient with a history of previous upper midline incision. *E* additional trocar used to take down adhesions; *C* insertion of the first camera port using a Hasson technique to the right of the umbilicus; *A* subxyphoid port; *B* midclavicular port; *D* retractor for gallbladder fundus. *S* surgeon; *CA* camera assistant; *FA* first assistant

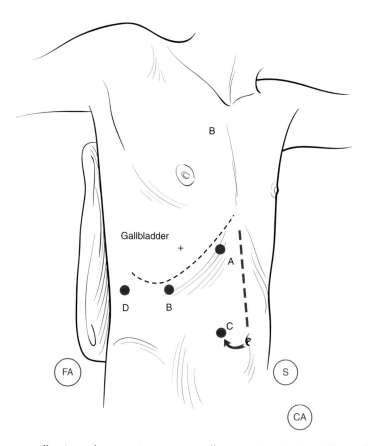

Fig. 2.15 Severe adhesions due to prior upper midline incision. Patient tilted after positioning on a bean bag. Camera (**c**) moved to the right and above the umbilical level. All other trocars (**a, b, d**) moved to the right

Agarwal BB (2009) Patient safety in laparoscopic cholecystectomy. Arch Surg 144(10):979

Baraka A, Jabbour S, Hammoud R et al (1994) End carbon dioxide tension during laparoscopic cholecystectomy, Correlation with the baseline value prior to carbon dioxide insuffiation. Anaesthesia 49(4):304–306

Bablekos GD, Michaelides SA, Roussou T, Charalabopoulos KA (2006) Changes in breathing control and mechanics after laparoscopic vs open cholecystectomy. Arch Surg 141(1):16–22

Barton JR, Russell RC, Hatfield AR (1995) Management of bile leaks after laparoscopic cholecystectomy. Br J Surg 82(7):980–984

Con P, Tate JJ, Lau WY, Dawson JW, Li AK (1994) Preoperative ultrasound to predict technical difficulties and complications of laparoscopic cholecystectomy. Am J Surg 168(1):54–56

Cushieri A, Dubois F, Mouiel J et al (1991) The European experience with laparoscopic cholecystectomy. Am J Surg 161:385–387

Davidoff AM, Pappas TN, Murray EA et al (1992) Mechanisms of major biliary injury during laparoscopic cholecystectomy. Ann Surg 215:196–202

Eisenstein S, Greenstein AJ, Kim U, Divino CM (2008) Cystic duct stump leaks: after the learning curve. Arch Surg 143(12):1178–1183

Essen P, Thorell A, McNurlan MA et al (1995) Laparoscopic cholecystectomy does not prevent the postoperative protein catabolic response in muscle. Ann Surg 222(1):36–42

Fabiani P, Iovine L, Katkhouda N, Gugenheim J, Mouiel J (1993) Dissection of the triangle of Calot during laparoscopic cholecystectomy. La Presse Medicale 22:535–537

Fenster LF, Lonborg R, Thirlby RC, Traverso LW (1995) What symptoms does cholecystect omy cure? Insights from an outcomes measurement project and review of the literature. Am J Surg 169(5):533–538

Fredman B, Jedeikin R, Olsfanger D, Flor P, Gruzman A (1994) Residual pneumoperitoneum: a cause of postoperative pain after laparoscopic cholecystecomy. Anesth Analg 79(1):152–154

Freeman JA, Armstrong IR (1994) Pulmonary function tests before and after laparoscopic cholecystectomy. Anaesthesia 49(7):579–582

Fried GM, Barkun JS, Sigman HH et al (1994) Factors determining conversion to laparotomy in patients undergoing laparoscopic cholecystectomy. Am J Surg 167(1):35–41

Fullarton GM, Darling K, Williams J, MacMillan R, Bell G (1994) Evaluation of the cost of laparoscopic and open cholecystectomy. Br J Surg 81(1):124–126

Glaser F, Sannwald GA, Buhr HJ et al (1995) General stress response to conventional and lapafoscopic cholecystectomy. Ann Surg 221(4):372–380

Glerup H, Heindorff H, Flyvbjerg A, Jensen SL, Vilstrup H (1995) Elective laparoscopic cholecystectomy nearly abolishes the postoperative hepatic catabolic stress response. Ann Surg 221(3):214–219

Gold-Deutch R, Mashiach R, Boldur I et al (1996) How does infected bile affect the post operative course of patients undergoing laparoscopic cholecystectomy? Am J Surg 172(3):272–274

Greig JD, John TG, Mahadaven M, Garden OJ (1994) Laparoscopic ultrasonography in the evaluation of the biliary tree during laparoscopic cholecystectomy. Br J Surg 81(8): 1202–1206

Halevy A, Gold-Deutch R, Negri M et al (1994) Are elevated liver enzymes and bilirubin levels significant after laparoscopic cholecystectomy in the absence of bile duct injury? Ann Surg 219(4):362–364

Jatzko GR, Lisborg PH, Perti AM, Stettner HM (1995) Multivariate comparison of complica tions after laparoscopic cholecystectomy and open cholecystectomy. Ann Surg 221(4):381–386

Jones DB, Dunnegan DL, Soper NJ (1995) Results of a change to routine fluorocholangiography during laparoscopic cholecystectomy. Surgery 118(4):693–701

Katkhouda N, Mavor E, Mason RJ (2000) Visual identification of the cystic duct–CBD junction during laparoscopic cholecystectomy (visual cholangiography). Surg Endosc 14:88–89

Kendall AP, Bhatt S, Oh TE (1995) Pulmonary consequences of carbon dioxide insufflation for laparoscopic cholecystectomies. Anaesthesia 50(4):286–289

Koo KP, Thirlby RC (1996) Laparoscopic cholecystectomy in acute cholecystitis. What is the optimal timing for operation? Arch Surg 131(5):540–544

Korman J, Cosgrove I, Furman M, Nathan I, Cohen J (1996) The role of endoscopic retrograde cholangiopancreatography and cholangiography in the laparoscopic era. Ann Surg 223(2):212–216

Kubota K, Bandai Y, Sano K, Teruya M, Ishizaki Y, Makuuchi M (1995) Appraisal of intraoperative ultrasonography during laparoscopic cholecystectomy. Surgery 118(3):555–561

Kuy S, Roman SA, Desai R, Sosa JA (2009) Outcomes following cholecystectomy in pregnant and nonpregnant women. Surgery 146(2):358–366

Lanzafame RI (1995) Laparoscopic cholecystectomy during pregnancy. Surgery 118(4): 627–631

Liu CL, Fan ST, Lai EC, Lo CM, Chu KM (1996) Factors affecting conversion of laparoscopic cholecystectomy to open surgery. Arch Surg 131(1):98–101

Lorimer JW, Fairfull-Smith RJ (1995) Intraoperative cholangiography is not essential to avoid duct injuries during laparoscopic cholecystectomy. Am J Surg 169(3):344–347

McLean TR (2006) Risk management observations from litigation involving laparoscopic cholecystectomy. Arch Surg 141(7):643–648

McMahon AS, Baxter JN, Murray W, Imrie CW, Kenny G, ODwyer PJ (1994) Helium pneumoperitoneum for laparoscopic cholecystectomy: ventilatory and blood gas changes. Br J Surg 81(7):1033–1036

Madariaga JR, Dodson SF, Selby R, Todo S, Iwatsuki S, Starzl TE (1994) Corrective treatment and anatomic considerations for laparoscopic cholecystectomy injuries. Am Coll Surg 179(3):321–325

Morgan RA, van Sonnenberg E, Wittich GR, Nealon WH, Walser EM (1995) Percutaneous management of bile duct injury after laparoscopic cholecystectomy. Am J Roentgenol 165(4):985–990

Nebiker CA, Frey DM, Hamel CT, Oertli D, Kettelhack C (2009) Early versus delayed cholecystectomy in patients with biliary acute pancreatitis. Surgery 145(3):260–264

Ortega AE, Peters JH, Incarbone R et al (1996) A prospective randomized comparison of the metabolic and stress hormonal responses of laparoscopic and open cholecystectomy. J Am Coll Surg 183(3):249–256

Perissat S, Huibregtse K, Keane PB, Russell RC, Neoptolemos JP (1994) Management of bile duct stones in the era of laparoscopic cholecystectomy. Br J Surg 81(6):799–810

Pertsemlidis D (2009) Fluorescent indocyanine green for imaging of bile ducts during laparoscopic cholecystectomy. Arch Surg 144(10):978

Peters JH, Krailadsiri W, Incarbone R et al (1994) Reasons for conversion from laparoscopic to open cholecystectomy in an urban teaching hospital. Am J Surg 168(6):555–559

Pietrabissa A, Di Candio G, Giulianotti PC, Shimi SM, Cuschieri A, Mosca F (1995) Comparative evaluation of contact ultrasonography and transcystic cholangiography during laparo scopic cholecystectomy: a prospective study. Arch Surg 130(10): 1110–1114

Ponce J, Cutshall KE, Hodge MJ, Browder W (1995) The lost laparoscopic stone. Potential for long-term complications. Arch Surg 130(6):666–668

Redmond HP, Watson RW, Houghton T et al (1994) Immune function in patients undergoing open vs laparoscopic cholecystectomy. Arch Surg 129(12):1240–1246

Robinson BL, Donohue JH, Gunes S et al (1995) Selective operative cholangiography. Appropriate management for laparoscopic cholecystectomy. Arch Surg 130(6):625–631

Roush TS, Traverso LW (1995) Management and long-term follow-up of patients with positive cholangiograms during laparoscopic cholecystectomy. Am J Surg 169(5):484–487

Sanabria JR, Gallinger S, Croxford R, Strasberg SM (1994) Risk factors in elective laparoscopic cholecystectomy for conversion to open cholecystectomy. Am Coll Surg 179(6):696–704

Savader SI, Lillemoe KD, Prescott CA et al (1997) Laparoscopic cholecystectomy-related bile duct injuries: a health and financial disaster. Ann Surg 225(3):268–273

Singh S, Agarwal AK (2009) Gallbladder cancer: the role of laparoscopy and radical resection. Ann Surg 250(3):494–495

Soper NJ, Brunt LM, Callery MP, Edmundowicz SA, Aliperti G (1994) Role of laparoscopic cholecystectomy in the management of acute gallstone pancreatitis. Am J Surg 167(1):42–50

The Southern Surgeons Club (1991) A prospective analysis of 1518 laparoscopic cholecystectomies. N Engl J Med 324:1073–1078

Strasberg SM (2008) Acute calculous cholecystitis. N Engl J Med 358(26):2804–2811

Steiner CA, Bass EB, Talamini MA, Pitt HA, Steinberg EP (1994) Surgical rates and operative mortality for open and laparoscopic cholecystectomy in Maryland. N Engl J Med 330(6):403–408

Stewart L, Way LW (1995) Bile duct injuries during laparoscopic cholecystectomy. Factors that influence the results of treatment. Arch Surg 130(10):1123–1129

Tate JJ, Lau WY, Li AK (1994) Laparoscopic cholecystectomy for biliary pancreatitis. Br J Surg 81(5):720–722

Teefy SA, Soper NJ, Middleton WD et al (1995) Imaging of the common bile duct during laparoscopic cholecystectomy: sonography versus videofluoroscopic cholangiography. Am J Roentgenol 165(4):847–851

Voyles CR, Sanders DL, Hogan R (1994) Common bile duct evaluation in the era of laparoscopic cholecystectomy. 1050 cases later. Ann Surg 219(6):744–752

Willekes CL, Edoga IK, Castronuovo JJ Jr, Widmann WD, McLean ER Jr, Chevinsky AH (1995) Technical elements of successful laparoscopic cholangiography as defined by radiographic criteria. Arch Surg 130(4):398–400

Woods MS, Traverso LW, Kozarek RA et al (1994a) Characteristics of biliary tract complications during laparoscopic cholecystectomy: a multi-institutional study. Am J Surg 167(1):27–34

Woods MS, Shellito JL, Santoscoy GS et al (1994b) Cystic duct leaks in laparoscopic cholecystectomy. Am J Surg 168(6):56–65

Yaghoubian A, Saltmarsh G, Rosing DK, Lewis RJ, Stabile BE, de Virgilio C (2008) Decreased bile duct injury rate during laparoscopic cholecystectomy in the era of the 80-hour resident workweek. Arch Surg 143(9):847–851

Yamaguchi K, Chijiiwa K, Ichimiya H et al (1996) Gallbladder carcinoma in the era of laparoscopic cholecystectomy. Arch Surg 131(9):981–985

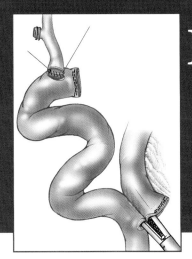

Common Bile Duct Explorations and Bilioenteric Anastomosis

3

Ｉf a stone is visualized during an intraoperative cholangiogram, a few measures should be attempted before proceeding to common bile duct (CBD) exploration. First, place the patient in steep reverse Trandelenberg and flush the CBD with saline. Intravenous Glucagon at a dose of 1 mg can also be given to relax the sphincter of Oddi and help the stone pass. If this is not successful, then one can proceed to a CBD exploration.

The Transcystic Approach

The transcystic approach is usually accepted as the initial approach in a CBD exploration. In this author's experience, the transcystic approach is a difficult maneuver that has not had the 95% success rate that some other authors have reported, and requires training.

The first step is to place an additional trocar directly above the cystic duct. This trocar will facilitate access to the cystic duct in a linear fashion. Next the cystic duct should be dilated by one of the following methods: inserting Maryland forceps into the duct, or using a dilating balloon, biliary Fogarty, or even stents of different calibers.

The next step is the insertion of a Dormia wire basket to retrieve the stones. This may be attempted without fluoroscopic guidance because the stones have already been located by intraoperative cholangiography. However, if retrieval of the stones proves difficult, then fluoroscopic guidance can be called upon before resorting to a choledochoscope. If the choledochoscope is needed to locate the stones, they can be removed using a wire basket introduced through the choledochoscope operating channel. If all these techniques are not successful, it will be necessary to revert to a laparoscopic choledochotomy.

N. Katkhouda, *Advanced Laparoscopic Surgery*,
DOI: 10.1007/978-3-540-74843-4_3, © Springer-Verlag Berlin Heidelberg 2011

The Common Bile Duct Approach

The first step is dissection of the CBD, as in open surgery, and this is done using very fine instruments in the right hand and an atraumatic grasper in the left hand. The peritoneal adhesions above the CBD are grasped with the left hand and the scissors are then used to peel these adhesions from the CBD. Peeling of the entire CBD is not indicated, as there is a risk of devascularizing the duct. Only an area appropriate for the choledochotomy is dissected out. Sharp micro-scissors are inserted and a choledochotomy is performed longitudinally. The size of the choledochotomy should be appropriate for the size of the CBD. *It should also match the size of the stone.* The same technique as in open surgery then applies, with the introduction of a choledochoscope with a 2.8 French channel into the midclavicular port to locate the stones. Introduction of the wire basket, either directly into the choledochotomy or via the operating channel of the laparoscope, will usually allow extraction of the stones from the CBD under direct vision. If a flexible choledochoscope is unavailable or stone removal by this method proves difficult, a traditional rigid choledochoscope can be introduced into the subxyphoid skin incision after removal of the 10 mm trocar. A suture can be tightened around the choledochoscope to keep the abdomen airtight. This can also be done directly through a separate skin incision. When the CBD has been cleared of all stones, it should be closed around a T-tube (Fig. 3.1). This T-tube is introduced through a separate small skin incision, and adequate tube length should be left in the abdomen in order to avoid its inadvertent dislodgement if an ileus is encountered postoperatively. The T-tube is cut to the appropriate size and inserted in the choledochotomy (Fig. 3.2). As in open surgery, it should be moved up and down to make sure that it is properly in place in the CBD. 4–0 PDS suture is used to close the choledochotomy in either an interrupted or continuous fashion, depending on the size of the CBD. Interrupted sutures tied intracorporeally are best for thin CBDs, while continuous

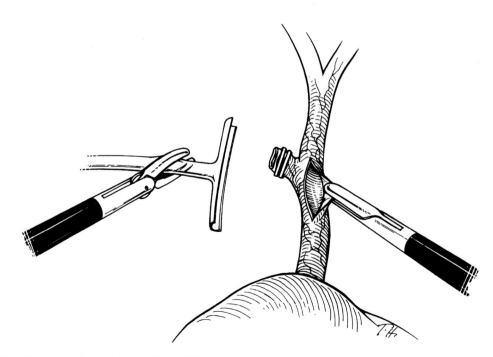

Fig. 3.1 Insertion of the T-tube in CBD exploration

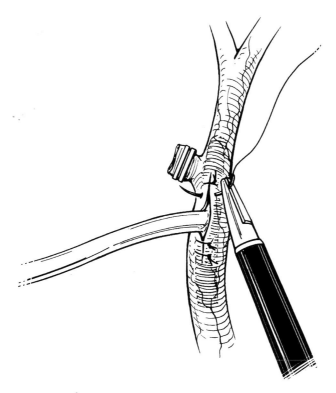

Fig. 3.2 Closure of the choledochotomy using 4–0 PDS

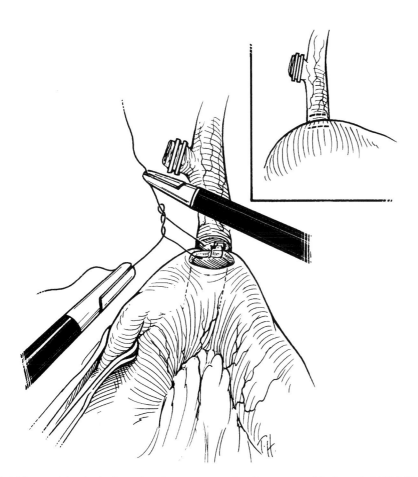

Fig. 3.3 Side-to-side choledocoduodenostomy using interrupted 3–0 or 4–0 PDS (full thickness on the posterior duodenal wall, extramucosal on the anterior duodenal wall)

sutures can be used on larger, dilated CBDs. Extracorporeal knot-tying is not useful in this setting. The T-tube is then tested for leaks by injecting some saline, before being properly fixed to the skin. A completion cholangiogram is performed. A drain is always inserted adjacent to the choledochotomy to monitor bile leakage.

Choledochodu-odenostomy

This procedure is similar to open surgery except that the choledochotomy should be performed transversely. The duodenum is then approximated and incised. Interrupted sutures are placed and knotted intracorporeally to avoid tension that might occur if they were to be knotted extracorporeally. Running sutures are possible if the CBD is very dilated.

The ideal suture is 3–0 PDS and square knots are tied using standard techniques (Fig. 3.3). The key to success is proper mobilization of the duodenum. This can be achieved easily by a partial Kocher maneuver of the duodenum. A drain should be left in place.

Hepaticoje-junostomy with a Roux-en-Y

This is a very difficult operation that should be attempted only by highly skilled laparo-scopic surgeons. The operative details are provided here for the reader's interest, rather than for absolute guidance. Six ports are used, as shown in Fig. 3.4. The operation starts with dissection of the CBD and separation from the important structures of the porta

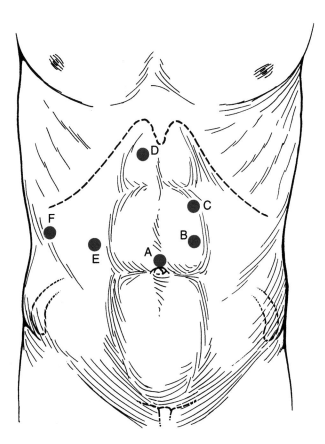

Fig. 3.4 Trocar port placement for laparoscopic hepaticojejunostomy. *A* umbilical laparo-scope; *B* surgeon's right hand (operating port); *C* irrigation suction probe; *D* liver fan retractor; *E* surgeon's left hand (grasper); *F* grasper (first assistant)

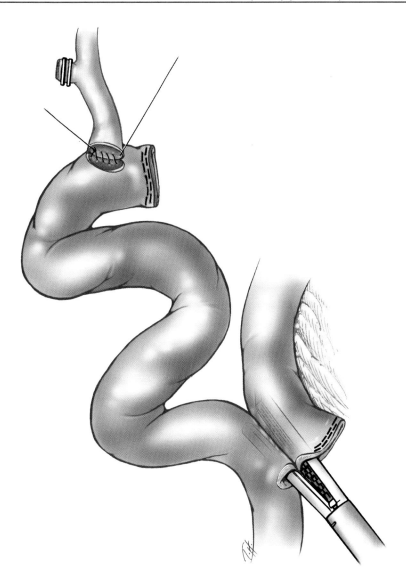

Fig. 3.5 End-to-side hepaticojejunostomy

hepatis, such as the hepatic artery and portal vein. It is important to use an atraumatic dissector very gently and to stay close to the CBD, using the magnification of the laparoscope as much as possible.

The CBD is encircled and umbilical tape is passed around it to allow gentle retraction of the duct. It is then transected. The distal end is ligated using an Endoloop with 2–0 PDS. The proximal end of the CBD is trimmed conservatively, care being taken to avoid devascularization. One then proceeds to prepare the Roux-en-Y loop (Fig. 3.5).

First the angle of Treitz is identified. Following the small bowel, the second jejunal loop is picked up and transection of the loop is performed using an EndoLinear Cutter-45 with white loads (Ethicon EndoSurgery Inc, Cincinatti, OH). One and half firings of the GIA-45 whites divide the mesentery. One should never fire more than two loads of 45-mm cutters in the mesentery to avoid injuring the superior mesenteric artery. The next step is coagulation of any bleeding along the cut edges of the mesentery. It is extremely important to perform this coagulation either by using electrocautery, or clips to avoid any postoperative bleeding. The harmonic shears are utilized to open up the crotch of this division to further enhance the length of the alimentary loop. Next a 40–60 cm Roux limb is selected and a jejunojejunostomy is performed after opening the proximal and distal limbs with the harmonic scalpel and then firing the 45 mm stapler with white loads. The enterotomy is closed with a running 3–0 Prolene in an extramucosal fashion. The mesentery defect is closed with nonabsorbable running suture. The Roux limb is then brought up and approximated to the end of the CBD. An enterotomy is performed, followed by creation of an anastomosis using a continuous suture on the posterior aspect of the jejunal wall. An interrupted 3–0 PDS is used on the anterior jejunal wall, ensuring the avoidance of the stricture of the hepatic duct.

Acosta J, Katkhouda N, Debian K, Groshen S, Berne TV (2006) Early ductal decompression vs conservative management for gallstone pancreatitis with ampullary obstruction. A prospective randomized trial. Ann Surg 243:33–40

Barkun AN, Barkun IS, Fried GM et al (1994) Useful predictors of bile duct stones in patients undergoing laparoscopic cholecystectomy. McGill Gallstone Treatment Group. Ann Surg 220(1):32–39

Barwood NT, Valinsky LJ, Hobbs MS, Fletcher DR, Knuiman MW, Ridout SC (2002) Changing methods of imaging the common bile duct in the laparoscopic cholecystectomy era in Western Australia: implications for surgical practice. Ann Surg 235(1):41–50

Berci G, Morgenstern L (1994) Laparoscopic management of common bile duct stones. A multi- institutional SAGES study. Society of American Gastrointestinal Endoscopic Surgeons. Surg Endosc 8(10):1168–1174

Carroll BJ, Phillips EH, Rosenthal R, Liberman M, Fallas M (1996) Update on transcystic exploration of the bile duct. Surg Laparosc Endosc 6(6):453–458

Crist DW, Davoudi MM, Parrino PE, Gadacz TR (1994) An experimental model for laparoscopic common bile duct exploration. Surg Laparosc Endosc 4(5):336–339

Croce E, Golia M, Azzola M et al (1996) Laparoscopic choledochotomy with primary closure. Follow-up (5–44 months) of 31 patients. Surg Endosc 10(11):1064–1068

DePaula AL, Hashiba K, Bafutto M (1994) Laparoscopic management of choledocholithiasis. Surg Endosc 8(12):1399–1403

de Reuver PR, Rauws EA, Bruno MJ, Lameris JS, Busch OR, van Gulik TM, Gouma DJ (2007) Survival in bile duct injury patients after laparoscopic cholecystectomy: a multidisciplinary approach of gastroenterologists, radiologists, and surgeons. Surgery 142(1):1–9

Fabiani P, Katkhouda N, Mouiel J (1987) Biliary lithiasis – clinical forms and treatment. Revue de l'étudiant de médecine 12:16–18 (in French)

Franklin ME Jr, Pharand D, Rosenthal D (1994) Laparoscopic common bile duct exploration. Surg Laparosc Endosc 4(2):119–124

Hugan SM, Wu CW, Chau GY, Jwo SC, Lui WY, Peng FK (1996) An alternative approach of choledocholithotomy: laparoscopic choledochotomy. Arch Surg 131(4):407–411

Martin IJ, Bailey IS, Rhodes M, O'Rourke N, Nathanson L, Fielding G (1998) Towards T-tube free laparoscopic bile duct exploration: a methodologic evolution during 300 consecutive procedures. Ann Surg 228(1):29–34

Miller RE, Kimmelstiel FM, Winkler WP (1995) Management of common bile duct stones in the era of laparoscopic cholecystectomy. Am J Surg 169(2):273–276

Moore DE, Feurer ID, Holzman MD, Wudel LJ, Strickland C, Gorden DL, Chari R, Wright JK, Pinson CW (2004) Long-term detrimental effect of bile duct injury on health-related quality of life. Arch Surg 139(5):476–481

Ponsky JL (1996) Endoscopic approaches to common bile duct injuries. Surg Clin N Am 76(3):505–513

Poulose BK, Speroff T, Holzman MD (2007) Optimizing choledocholithiasis management: a cost-effectiveness analysis. Arch Surg 142(1):43–48

Robertson US, Jagger C, Johnson PR et al (1996) Selection criteria for preoperative endoscopic retrograde cholangiopancreatography in the laparoscopic era. Arch Surg 131(1):89–94

Sarmiento JM, Farnell MB, Nagorney DM, Hodge DO, Harrington JR (2004) Quality-of-life assessment of surgical reconstruction after laparoscopic cholecystectomy-induced bile duct injuries: what happens at 5 years and beyond? Arch Surg 139(5):483–488

Stoker ME (1995) Common bile duct exploration in the era of laparoscopic surgery. Arch Surg 130(3):265–269

Tang E, Stain SC, Tang G, Froes B, Berne TV (1995) Timing of laparoscopic surgery in gallstone pancreatitis. Arch Surg 130(5):496–500

Tekin A, Ogetman Z, Altunel E (2008) Laparoendoscopic "rendezvous" versus laparoscopic antegrade sphincterotomy for choledocholithiasis. Surgery 144(3):442–447

Tinoco R, Tinoco A, El-Kadre L, Peres L, Sueth D (2008) Laparoscopic common bile duct exploration. Ann Surg 247(4):674–679

Walsh RM, Henderson JM, Vogt DP, Brown N (2007) Long-term outcome of biliary reconstruction for bile duct injuries from laparoscopic cholecystectomies. Surgery 142(4): 450–456

Laparoscopic Liver Surgery

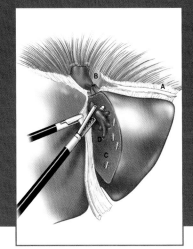

4

With appropriate patient selection and proper equipment, laparoscopic liver surgery can take place with relative comfort and safety. Patient selection will be discussed briefly at the end of the chapter.

The Need for Specialized Equipment

In addition to the standard instruments described in Chap. 1, it is necessary to have instruments specifically adapted to hepatic surgery. High-quality 30-degree and even 45-degree laparoscopes should be available.

Forceps used on the liver should be flat and atraumatic, without teeth. All the forceps should be insulated, with rotating capability. It is also desirable to have rotating coagulation scissors, and hooks that are entirely insulated at the tip. A spatula is important for hemostasis on flat surfaces. One should only proceed with automatic clip appliers that allow clips to be placed without withdrawing the instrument for reloading. Stapling devices with vascular white cartridges are extremely useful for control of certain vascular pedicles.

Other specific instruments include the argon-beam coagulator, ultrasonic dissectors, laparoscopic ultrasound, and harmonic scissors.

Harmonic shears are also very useful tools in liver surgery. The lower blades oscillate at 55,000 Hz, generating localized heat and coagulation of proteins. It serves as a welding tool and is ideal for hemostasis of smaller vessels. Laparoscopic ultrasound probes are useful especially when coupled with color Doppler. They can help determine the limits and vascular involvement of solid masses, which is critical when a tumor is posterior and dangerously close to the inferior vena cava or the origins of hepatic veins. Fibrin glue (Tisseal, Baxter Inc, Deerfield Il) is used and can be very efficient in achieving complete hemostasis after laparoscopic hepatic resection. Its ideal application is on a decapsulated, dry liver surface. Adhesive fibrin sealant is available in various concentrations and with

N. Katkhouda, *Advanced Laparoscopic Surgery*,
DOI: 10.1007/978-3-540-74843-4_4, © Springer-Verlag Berlin Heidelberg 2011

various coagulation times. It should be applied without pressure to the raw surfaces of the liver at the end of the resection. Floseal (Baxter Inc, Deerfield IL) is another hemostatic agent in a granular form well adapted to achieve hemostasis crevices and deeper liver breaks. Omentum can then be applied to achieve an omentoplasty. Biliary ducts should be ligated with absorbable monofilament thread (3–0 and 4–0 PDS) and vascular structures can be ligated with silk ties. Specimen retrieval bags must be strong and equipped with a closing system.

Positioning the Patient and Operating Team

The author prefers to stand in the French position (see Fig. 1.1b). The surgeon stands between the patient's lower limbs, which are spread and placed in sequential compression devices on padded supports to avoid deep venous thrombosis and pressure necrosis. This arrangement is comfortable for the surgeon, who does not have to bend unnecessarily, which may occur when he or she is standing to the side, and it provides a symmetric view of the monitors. This position is also convenient for the assistants on each side.

The monitors are placed on each side of the anesthesiologist near the head of the patient. The scrub technician stands to the right of the surgeon, beside the camera assistant, allowing him or her to pass instruments to the surgeon's right hand. All traditional instruments for open surgery must be at hand in case immediate conversion becomes necessary. The usual rules of anesthesiology for hepatic surgery are followed, but the anesthesiologist must be aware of the additional hazards of laparoscopic liver surgery, such as a potential CO_2 embolism or massive perioperative bleeding. Sufficient supplies of plasma and blood must be readily available.

Access to the Liver

A minimum of four ports must be introduced for basic liver procerdures (beyond simple diagnostic laproscopy). The ports are placed to allow enough space between them to avoid the knitting needle effect between the various instruments. The port for the laparoscope is usually introduced at the umbilicus, the port for the graspers on the right side, and the port for the operating instruments on the left side of the patient. This triangle is enlarged to a rectangle by placing a fourth port for palpation and/or the irrigation/aspiration probe (Fig. 4.1a, b). This arrangement can be varied according to the location of the lesion and the working method to which the surgeon is accustomed; there is no "ideal" arrangement of the ports for this type of surgery.

All ports must be at least 10 mm to allow the camera to be moved from port to port to visualize the hepatic lesion from different angles. Further trocars can be introduced for specific instruments – five or six is realistically the maximum number of trocars if the operating field is not to be overcrowded. This allows two surgeons to perform simultaneously with a "four-handed" approach (Fig. 4.2a). One surgeon manipulates a grasper and dissects with the CUSA while the other surgeon is needed to divide using clips and scissors. This four handed approach minimizes hemorrhage and speeds up the procedure (Fig. 4.2b).

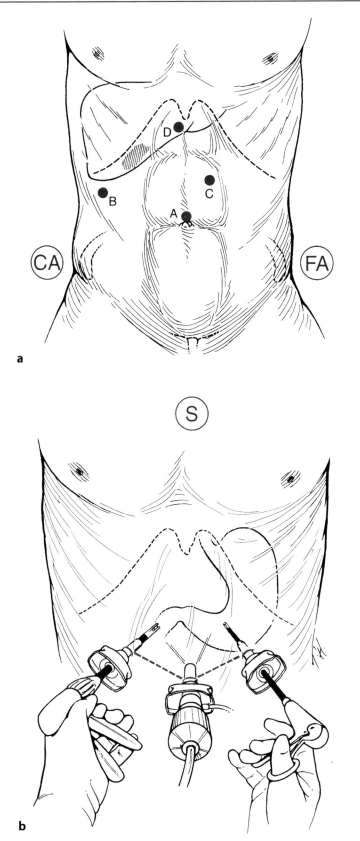

Fig. 4.1 (**a**) Port placement for basic liver procedures. *A* umbilical scope; *B* surgeon's left hand; *C* surgeon's right hand; *D* suction irrigation device or for retraction. *S* surgeon standing between the left; *FA* first assistant; *CA* camera assistant. (**b**) Port placement for basic liver procedures. The triangulation concept

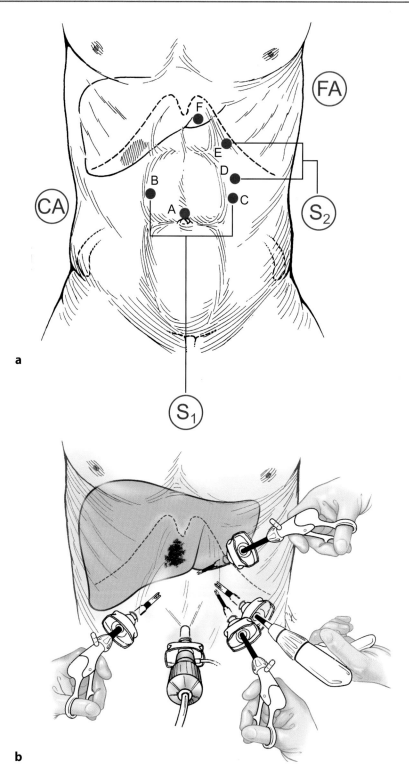

Fig. 4.2 (**a**) Port placement for advanced liver procedures (resection) using the "four hands approach." *A* laparoscope; *B* main surgeon's left hand (grasper); *C* main surgeon's right hand (harmonic shears); *D* second surgeon's left hand (grasper or scissors); *E* second surgeon's right hand (clip applier); *F* suction irrigation device or fan retractor. *S1* first surgeon; *S2* second surgeon; *FA* first assistant; *CA* camera assistant. (**b**) Four hands approach during liver resection

As with open surgery, laparoscopic surgery starts with mobilization of the liver (Fig. 4.3). This is the key to successful surgery as it clears the area surrounding the lesion allowing direct access. This procedure is familiar to all hepatic surgeons.

The first step is division and ligation of the round and falciform ligaments between clips, with a vascular stapler, or with the harmonic shears so that the anterosuperior surface of the liver can be pushed down. Retraction of the liver is achieved with a fan retractor held by an assistant, while the surgeon brings the harmonic shears above the liver and divides the triangular ligament under direct view. The left triangular ligament is divided if the lesion is on the left lobe, or partial division of the right triangular ligament (which is more difficult) for a right posterior lesion. During a major resection, such as a left lateral segmentectomy, it is necessary to be able to approach the side of the superior vena cava to control the hepatic veins, in particular the left hepatic vein. Once the liver is completely mobilized an incision is made in Glisson's capsule, using the harmonic shears (Fig. 4.4).

Next, long Kelly forceps simulate the finger fracture method. An ultrasonic dissector is very handy here, enabling parenchymal destruction while preserving the vascular and ductal elements. All large vascular vessels must be controlled by clips or by ties in the case of a major vessel or biliary duct. Vascular endolinear cutters are extremely useful for controlling large vessels.

At the end of the operation, the liver segment must be placed in a suitable retrieval bag that allows extraction without spillage of liver cells. Extraction is usually accomplished by enlarging the umbilical opening. Other extraction sites are possible; for larger specimens, a suprapubic incision can be used, or in the case of hand-assisted techniques, the extraction site is the same as the incision used for the introduction of the gelport and the nondominant hand (depicted here on the right side of the patient, Fig. 4.5). The

Maneuvers Common to All Laparoscopic Liver Surgery

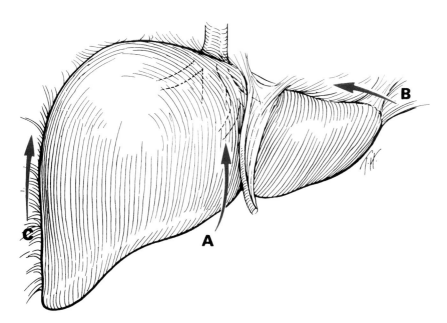

Fig. 4.3 Mobilization of the liver. *A* faliciform ligament; *B* left triangular ligament; *C* right triangular ligament

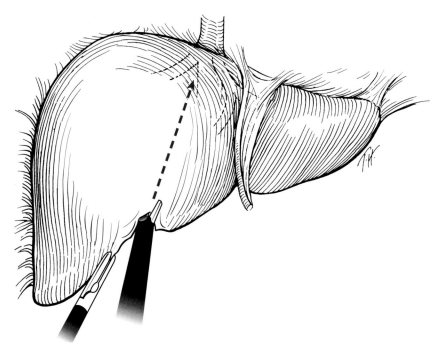

Fig. 4.4 Incision in Glisson's capsule using harmonic shears (initiation of the resection)

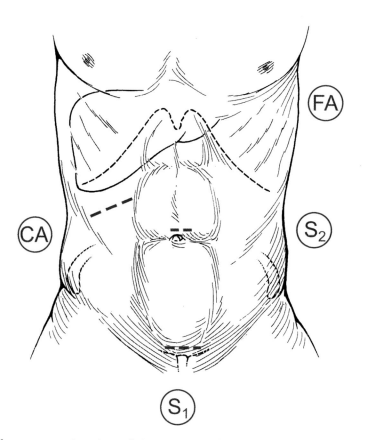

Fig. 4.5 Different extraction sites of the specimen for hand-assisted laparoscopic surgery (HALS): supraumbilical, suprapubic, or subcostal. *S1* main surgeon; *S2* second surgeon; *FA* first assistant

resected specimen can be *partially* morcelated with the Kelly forceps if a morcelator is not available. The liver specimen should never be reduced to a total mush, which would not allow postoperative pathological examination.

Diagnostic laparoscopy can be used to look for small tumors of the liver that may not be detectable by conventional imaging techniques. Pancreatic cancer, for example, is often accompanied by small multiple hepatic metastases that are spread throughout the entire organ. Because of their small size, these and other intraperitoneal seedings are sometimes undetectable by standard imaging methods, but can usually be seen with a laparoscope. This can change the indication from a curative resection to palliative surgery, or even to nonintervention in very advanced cases. Diagnostic laparoscopy is also useful in identifying liver involvement unseen by preoperative imaging in cancer of the gallbladder.

The diagnostic procedure involves a laparoscope introduced via an umbilical port, with another port to allow for biopsy.

Laparoscopic *ultrasonography* is a valuable technique for studying the liver. Users who have sufficient experience can produce images that are as helpful as images obtained by intraoperative open ultrasonography. Laparoscopic ultrasonography enables the detection of deeper lying metastases as well as underlying connections to vital structures such as the hepatic veins. The hepatic vessels as well as the biliary ducts can be seen clearly. With intraoperative ultrasonography, a biopsy can be directed without fear of causing major hemorrhaging or bile leaks.

Diagnostic Laparoscopy

This is a relatively easy procedure; for single giant cysts, the basic trocar approach is used (Fig. 4.1a, b). The harmonic shears are used to fenestrate the cyst after incising its most protuberant area. Each leaf of the cyst is elevated with the grasper, and the cyst is excised at its junction with normal hepatic parenchyma (Fig. 4.7). Clips should be placed to ensure hemostasis, as the number one postoperative problem is bleeding from the liver edge. If the cyst is very large with a thick membrane, a linear cutter with vascular loads can be used to achieve this resection at the liver edge. In the case of polycystic liver disease, the operation proceeds with the same technique through previously unroofed cysts; however, when dealing with deeper cysts, care should be exercised to avoid injury to a hepatic vein or pedicle, as these vascular structures have a similar appearance as that of liver cysts under the illumination of the laparoscope (transparent with a bluish tinge).

Fenestration of Liver Cysts
(Fig. 4.6)

Enucleation, wedge resection, anterior segmentectomies, and left lateral segmentectomies are reasonable laparoscopic technical possibilities. Lobectomies are very advanced procedures reserved for a few laparoscopic liver experts (Fig. 4.8).

Resection of Liver Tumors

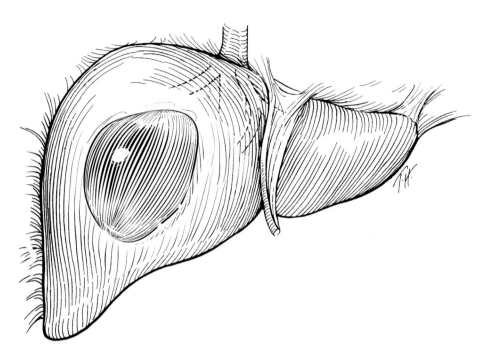

Fig. 4.6 Fenestration of liver cysts

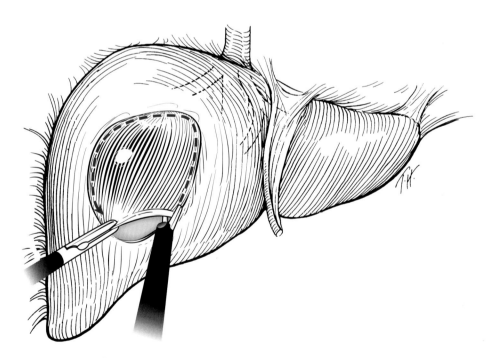

Fig. 4.7 Excision of cystic wall using harmonic shears

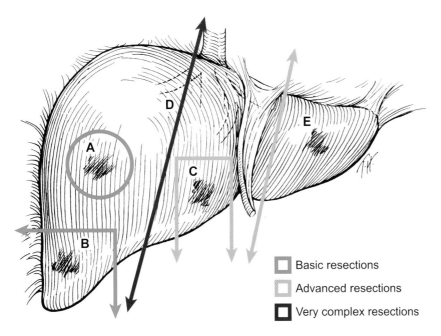

Fig. 4.8 Different levels of complexity based on learning curve. *A* enucleation; *B* atypical peripheral wedge; *C* segmentectomy; *E* left lateral sectoriectomy; *D* lobectomy

Limited Resection of Minor Lesions

Wedge resection of a solid benign tumor, such as an adenoma, is a good example of a small lesion that can be removed laparoscopically. A small metastasis in the left lobe also can be safely resected under laparoscopy with a reasonable 15–20 mm surgical margin. Four trocars are necessary for access: an umbilical trocar for the laparoscope, two large trocars for the grasping forceps and other instruments, and one sub-xiphoid trocar for the irrigation/aspiration probe. For a larger resection it is necessary to use the "four-handed approach" described above (Fig. 4.2a, b).

The resection begins with incision of Glisson's capsule 2 cm from the lesion. Smoke must be sucked out intermittently through the irrigation/aspiration cannula. It is then necessary to dissect progressively deeper into the hepatic parenchyma using the harmonic shears while separating the edges of the liver with the left handed forceps. Sometimes a fifth trocar is needed for the assistant to insert a grasper to carefully move the tumor mass. This will create a groove through which a hook or coagulating scissors can pass. Atraumatic grasping forceps allow the minute structures to be coagulated as they pass through this groove. All bile ducts should be clipped or tied; it is not recommended to rely on the harmonic shears to seal bile ducts, as this can lead to postoperative bile leaks. Clips must be employed for larger vessels, and it is recommended that a double clipping technique be used to avoid inadvertent dislocation of a single clip on a vascular pedicle. The irrigation/aspiration probe should be used in a deep groove in the liver to keep the operating field dry. The need to maintain a bloodless field by means of constant rinsing of the dissection area cannot be overemphasized. With a small wedge resection drainage is not usually necessary.

When dealing with large liver masses, the author routinely performs cholangiography at the conclusion of the resection, to identify possible biliary leaks. This, of course, cannot be done without cholecystectomy. A 5–8 cm solid tumor can be extracted in a bag without difficulty by enlarging the fascial incision at the umbilicus so that the extracted specimen is left intact. The specimen should always be removed in a *tumor-proof solid bag*.

Left Lateral Segmentectomy

This approach is aimed at larger tumors on the left lobe for which a wedge resection or limited segmentectomy may prove to be incomplete and therefore inadequate treatment. Larger lesions of the left lobe may also be best dealt with by a formal resection when a wedge procedure might actually prove to be more difficult and hazardous. Laparoscopic left lateral segmentectomy, however, should only be considered by surgeons who have extensive experience in both laparoscopy and liver surgery.

Placement of the ports is as shown in Fig. 4.2a, b. This allows for simultaneous maneuvers by two surgeons operating in harmony (four hands approach) - one doing the dissection and the other concentrating on hemostatic control and the clipping of all vessels. The lead surgeon usually operates the ultrasonic dissector while the second surgeon applies clips and divides the isolated vessels. This technique speeds the procedure and enhances safety.

The procedure follows the same rules as in open surgery. It begins with extremely careful hepatic vascular isolation. This includes the left hepatic vein which must be isolated before the liver capsule is incised. The falciform ligament is divided until the vena cava is seen.

A Pringle maneuver can then he performed using an atraumatic right-angled dissector, and a tourniquet is placed around the porta hepatis (Fig. 4.9a, b). Then, after full mobilization of the left triangular ligament, it is possible to retract the left lobe inferiorly using an atraumatic fan retractor allowing one to see the insertion of the left hepatic vein on the vena cava. *This is an extremely dangerous maneuver and should be done only by a very skilled laparoscopic surgeon.*

Now a right-angled atraumatic dissector is introduced and the left hepatic vein is encircled using gentle blunt dissection and a long tic placed around it. An atraumatic clamp should always be kept handy in the vicinity in case there is bleeding that requires immediate compression and clamping. However, a bleeding left hepatic vein is a dramatic event. Therefore, unless this vessel is safely controlled within seconds of hemorrhaging, the surgeon should opt for an immediate safe conversion. If the left hepatic vein has a short course outside the liver parenchyma before joining the inferior vena cava, dissection should not be attempted. The vein will be controlled during parenchymal dissection.

After incision of the capsule, dissection is continued into the deep parenchyma. During parenchymal dissection one encounters the constituents of the portal pedicle. They are ideally controlled with clips, and reinforced by intracorporeal ligatures when necessary. Intracorporeal knotting will avoid traction on the vessel. That said, it is easier to try to secure all vascular elements with clips, as it is difficult to apply sutures laparoscopically in the liver as the tissue is very friable.

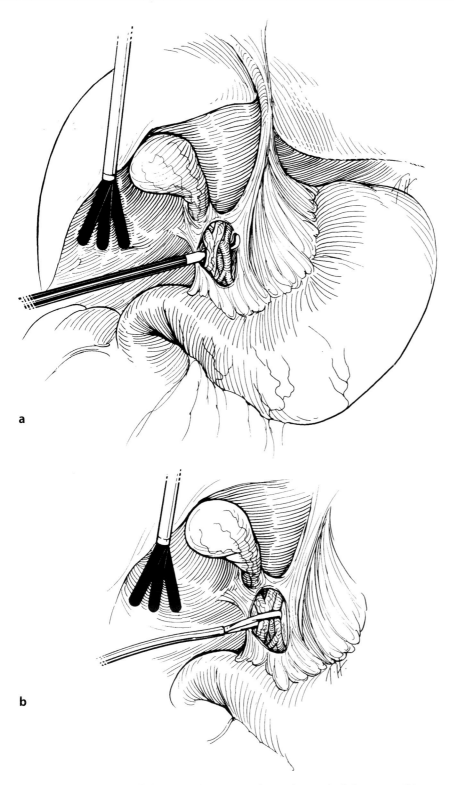

a

b

Fig. 4.9 (a) Dissection around the porta hepatis with a right-angled dissector. (**b**) Tourniquet around the porta hepatis using umbilical tape and a section of rubber tube

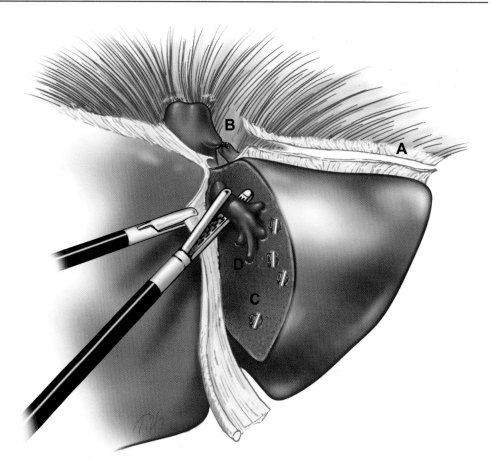

Fig. 4.10 Left lateral segmentectomy with intrahepatic division of the left hepatic vein. *A* division of left triangular ligament; *B* extrahepatic ligation of left hepatic vein; *C* control of vascular pedicles of segments II and III; *D* division of left hepatic vein

The last vessel to be encountered is the left hepatic vein that has been isolated previously. It is transected using a vascular stapler (Fig. 4.10).

In general, the lobectomy specimen is then placed in an extraction bag and can be withdrawn only if it undergoes some degree of morcelation. The hepatic surfaces are inspected and hemostasis is completed. Here again, cholangiographic examination to detect bile leaks is useful. The application of fibrin sealant when possible is invaluable. The greater omentum can be used to cover the raw surface of the liver at the end of the procedure. After left lateral segmentectomy, the procedure concludes with the placement of two suction drains near the edge of the wound to collect any minor persistent oozing of blood or bile and to prevent hematomas.

Smaller resections such as limited segmentectomies are done in the same way, with the same concern for hemostasis and control of the biliary ducts. One good method is to use vascular staplers for these minor liver resections. Vascular white staples can easily control the hemostasis of small pedicles but it is advisable to start the resection by scarring the capsule with a hook. Once the parenchyma is penetrated, the vascular stapler can then be applied.

Katkhouda N, Heimbucher J, Mills S, Mouiel J (1994) Management of problems in laparoscopic surgery of the biliary tract. Ann Chi Gynaecol 83:93–99

Katkhouda N (2008) Application of fibrin glue after hepatectomy might still be justified. Ann Surg 247(2):399–400

Katkhouda N, Hurwitz M, Gugenheim J, Mavor E, Mason RJ, Waldrep DJ, Rivera RT, Chandra M, Campos GM, Offerman S, Trussler A, Fabiani P, Mouiel J (1999b) Laparoscopic management of benign solid and cystic lesions of the liver. Ann Surg 229(4):460–466

Katkhouda N, Iovine L, Nano JL, Mouiel J (1993) A comparative study of ND-YAG laser and electrocautery for liver metastatic resection in the rat. Lasers Med Sci 38:55–62

Katkhouda N, Mouiel J (1992) Laser resection of a liver hydatid cyst by videocoelioscopy. Br J Surg 79:560–561

Katkhouda N, Fabiani P, Le Goff P, Mouiel J (1989a) Hepatic parameters as indicators of common bile duct stones. Lettre Chir 72:12–17

Katkhouda N, Tricarico A, Castillo L, Bertrandy M, Mouiel J (1989) Complications of external bile drainage in the surgery of extra-hepatic lithiasis. A general review of 156 cases. Chir Epatobiliare 10:5–9 (in Italian)

Libutti SK, Starker PM (1994) Laparoscopic resection of a nonparasitic liver cyst. Surg Endosc 8(9):1105–1107

Marks J, Mouiel J, Katkhouda N, Gugenhein J, Fabani P (1998) Laparoscopic liver surgery. A report on 28 patients. Surg Endosc 12:331–334

Morino M, DeGiuli M, Festa V, Garrone C (1994) Laparoscopic management of symptomatic nonparasitic cysts of the liver. Indications and results. Ann Surg 219(2):157–164

Mouiel J, Katkhouda N, Gugenheim J, Fabiani P (2000) Possibilities of laparoscopic liver resection. J Hepatobiliary Pancreatic Surg 7:1–8

Mouiel J, Katkhouda N, Fabiani P (1998) Complications of biliary lithiasis. Etiology, diagnosis, principals of drug therapy and surgery. Rev Prat 38(19):1309–1314

Nguyen KT, Laurent A, Dagher I, Geller DA, Steel J, Thomas MT, Marvin M, Ravindra KV, Mejia A, Lainas P, Franco D, Cherqui D, Buell JF, Gamblin TC (2009a) Minimally invasive liver resection for metastatic colorectal cancer: a multi-institutional, international report of safety, feasibility, and early outcomes. Ann Surg 250(5):842–848

Nguyen KT, Gamblin TC, Geller DA (2009b) World review of laparoscopic liver resection-2, 804 patients. Ann Surg 250(5):831–841

Ooi LL, Cheong LH, Mack PO (1994) Laparoscopic marsupialization of liver cysts. Aust NZ J Surg 64(4):262–263

Sato M, Watanabe Y, Ueda S, Kawachi K (1997) Minimally invasive hepatic resection using laparoscopic surgery and minithoracotomy. Arch Surg 132(2):206–208

Schob OM, Schlumpf RB, Tlhlschmid GK, Rausis C, Spiess M, Largiader F (1995) Experimental laparoscopic liver resection with a multimodal water jet dissector. Br J Surg 82(3):392–393

Shaughnessy TE, Raskin D (1995) Cardiovascular collapse after laparoscopic liver biopsy. Br J Anaesth 75(6):782–784

Tate JJ, Lau WY, Li AK (1994) Transhepatic fenestration of liver cyst: a further application of laparoscopic surgery. Aust NZ J Surg 64(4):264–265

Vigano L, Laurent A, Tayar C, Tomatis M, Ponti A, Cherqui D (2009) The learning curve in laparoscopic liver resection: improved feasibility and reproducibility. Ann Surg 250(5):772–782

Watanabe Y, Sato M, Ueda S et al (1997) Laparoscopic hepatic resection: a new and safe procedure by abdominal wall lifting method. Hepatogastroenterology 44(13):143–147

Esophageal Surgery 5

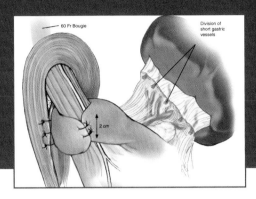

Principles of Surgical Therapy in the Management of Gastroesophageal Reflux Disease

Nissen Fundoplication

Surgery aims to achieve the following:

- Reduction of a hiatal hernia and resection of the sac if present
- Fixation of the lower esophageal sphincter in the abdomen, allowing it to function under positive intra-abdominal pressure
- Closure of the crura behind the esophagus to keep the wrap in the abdomen
- Ensuring an adequate length of the intra-abdominal sphincter
- Correcting the defective sphincter pressure while still allowing the sphincter to relax on swallowing.

Obtaining a fine balance of the sphincter pressure is critical to avoid postoperative complications such as dysphagia or gas bloating.

The technical goals are closure of the diaphragmatic crura behind the esophagus and fundoplication creating a short floppy wrap of 15–20 mm in length. Mobilization of the wrap is achieved by division of the short gastric vessels, and calibration of the wrap is performed around a 60 Fr bougie (Fig. 5.1).

Patient Positioning

The patient is placed in lithotomy position. The surgeon stands between the patient's legs with the monitor directly ahead. The first assistant stands to the surgeon's right and the camera assistant to the surgeon's left. The patient's arms are tucked (Fig. 5.2).

N. Katkhouda, *Advanced Laparoscopic Surgery*,
DOI: 10.1007/978-3-540-74843-4_5, © Springer-Verlag Berlin Heidelberg 2011

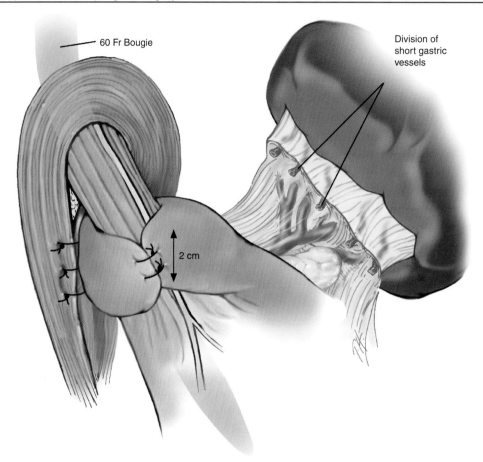

60 Fr Bougie

Division of
short gastric
vessels

2 cm

Fig. 5.1 "Gold standard Nissen" fundoplication according to DeMeester = short, floppy wrap calibrated around a 60 Fr bougie

The patient's pelvis should be secured to avoid sliding when in steep reverse Trendelenberg. It is important to make sure that the legs are extended to avoid conflict between the elbows of the surgeon and the knees of the patient, and to enable the surgeon to operate comfortably. As always, the patient should be carefully cushioned to prevent pressure injuries, and have sequential compression devices on to prevent deep vein thrombosis.

Technique

Pneumoperitoneum is established using a Veress needle inserted at the umbilicus. Once the usual security precautions have been performed using a 10 mL syringe, an incision is made to insert the first and most important port for the laparoscope. If this first port is inserted too low the surgeon will have only a flat horizontal view of the hiatus and the stomach will block the view. If the port is inserted too high on the midline, the surgeon will not have the necessary "panoramic view" to evaluate the entire operative field. The position of this port depends on the patient's habitus. *As a rule of thumb* the first port is inserted close to the midline at about two-thirds of the distance down between the xiphoid process and the umbilicus, and slightly to the left of the midline to avoid the falciform ligament.

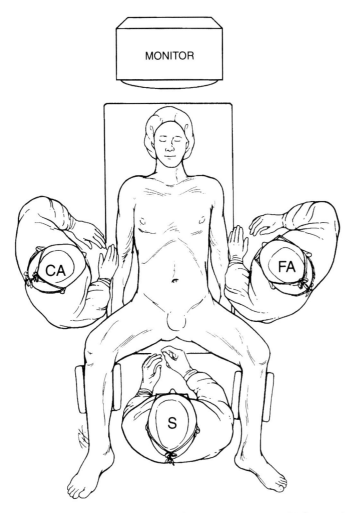

Fig. 5.2 Patient positioning for Nissen fundoplication. *S* surgeon; *FA* first assistant; *CA* camera assistant

The second 10–12 mm port is placed just under the xiphoid process, with care being taken to avoid branches of the superior epigastric vessels. This port will be used to introduce the liver retractor. The blunt round tip of the device affords less danger of traumatizing the left lobe, although a standard atraumatic fan retractor can be used.

The third port to be inserted is the right lateral one, for the grasping instruments in the surgeon's left hand. The fourth is the left lateral trocar used by the first assistant; this port is placed in line with the right lateral trocar, a few centimeters under the left costal margin. The fifth port is for the operating instruments in the surgeon's right hand and is placed midway between the video laparoscope and the left lateral trocar. All five ports are triangulated with one another to enable comfortable operation and form a diamond with extension to the left (Fig. 5.3).

When the ports have been inserted the operating table is placed in steep reverse Trendelenburg. This causes the stomach and other organs to fall away from the diaphragm, providing better access to the hiatus. The operation should be performed meticulously and with careful hemostasis to avoid obscuring the vision with blood or other fluids pooling under the diaphragm. Irrigation should thus be kept to a minimum.

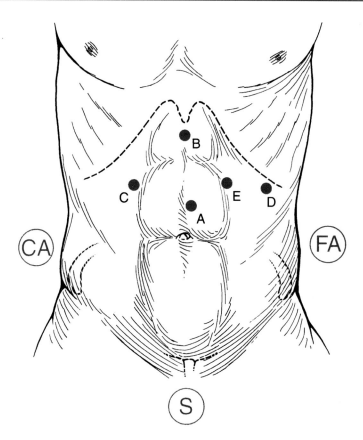

Fig. 5.3 Port positions for Nissen fundoplication. *A* supraumbilical laparoscope; *B* subxiphoid trocar for liver retractor; *C* grasper in surgeon's left hand; *D* grasper for first assistant; *E* operating port. *S* surgeon; *FA* first assistant; *CA* camera assistant

The steps of the procedure can be summarized as follows:

1) Access the hiatus by opening the avascular aspect of the lesser sac and preserving the hepatic branch of the left vagus nerve whenever possible.
2) Identification of the important landmarks that will lead to the hiatus; i.e., the caudate lobe to the right, and the right crus to the left of the caudate lobe.
3) Dissection between the esophagus and right crus in an avascular plane, and identification of the right vagus nerve.
4) Demonstration of the left crus from the right side (the left crus and the right crus form a V shape).
5) Creation of a retroesophageal window beginning below the left crus and under the esophagus.
6) Division of the phrenoesophageal membrane and the angle of His, preserving the branches of the left vagus nerve.
7) Demonstration of the left crus on the left side of the esophagus.
8) Completion of the window to allow the passage of the wrap and placement of a Penrose drain around the esophagus.
9) Division of the short gastric vessels starting at the mid fundus, and proceeding superiorly until the angle of His is encountered and the fundus can be flipped medially and the left crus is clearly seen behind the rolled fundus.

10) Reconstruction of a normal hiatus by closure of the crura behind the esophagus, creation of the wrap calibrated around a 60 Fr bougie by sliding the posterior fundus behind the esophagus and fixing it to the anterior fundus, the end result being a short 15–20 mm floppy wrap.

■ **Access to the Hiatus.** After retraction of the left lobe, the avascular aspect of the lesser sac is demonstrated and is exposed with the left hand using an atraumatic grasper without ratchets while the assistant exposes by retracting the stomach, giving more freedom for tissue manipulation (Fig. 5.4a). The harmonic shears are held in the right hand and used to divide the "window." Care is taken to preserve the hepatic branch of the left vagus when possible, although inadvertent division of this branch does not seem to have any postoperative consequences such as dumping, diarrhea, or increased incidence of gallbladder stones. Another important structure that may be encountered in this area is an accessory left hepatic artery, which can be clamped with an atraumatic grasper and then divided if there is no evidence of ischemia of the left lateral lobe.

One can now identify the caudate lobe on the right side, and just adjacent to the caudate lobe the pink color of the right crus will be visible (Fig. 5.4b). At this point the anesthesiologist is asked to mobilize the nasogastric tube, thus putting the esophagus on tension, helping to confirm its identification. The dissection is begun by grasping the right crus with an atraumatic grasper, and using the harmonic scalpel, an incision is made on the peritoneum overlying the right crus. This will lead to an avascular plane between the esophagus and the right crus. It is of paramount importance to stay on the right crus during this part of the dissection.

The plane is opened with a sweeping motion using laparoscopic Babcocks, and the posterior trunk of the vagus nerve can usually be found easily, either along the right side of the esophagus or running on the left crus. The posterior vagus can be identified by its white color and the small blue veins covering its surface. It is usually a large trunk and will resist attempts to tear it with a grasper. It is left in place, and no attempt should be made to dissect it off the esophagus to avoid devascularization.

■ **Identification of the Left Crus at the Right Side of the Esophagus.** This is one of the key elements of the procedure. Indeed, identification of the left crus at the right side of the esophagus will lead to a demonstration of the *crural V* shape decussation that will help the creation of a window under the esophagus used to bring the wrap around the esophagus (Fig. 5.5).

■ **Creation of a Window Under the Esophagus.** The window is created using a Babcock grasper. This requires a gentle opening and closing motion of the grasper's jaws behind the esophagus without ever fully grasping it. Another technique is a sweeping "breaststroke" motion of two atraumatic graspers. A space for the wrap is thus created below the left crus and posterior to the esophagus (Fig. 5.6). It is not necessary to completely dissect blindly behind the esophagus, but rather stop at this point and proceed to the next step.

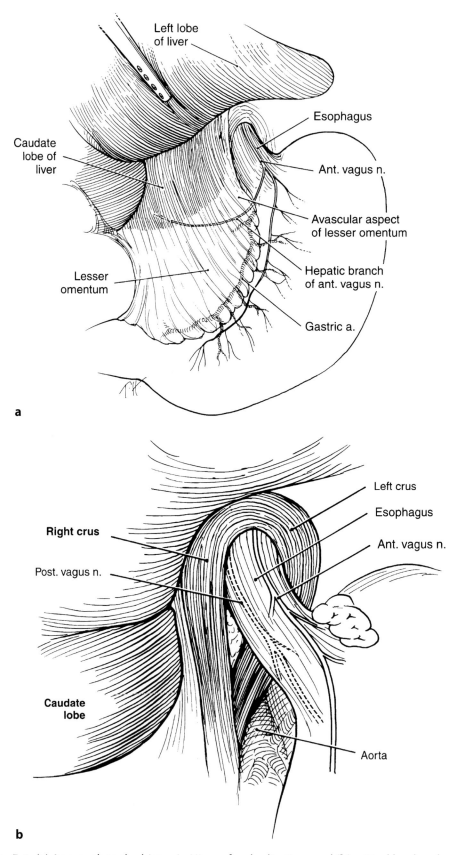

Fig. 5.4 (**a**) Approach to the hiatus in Nissen fundoplication, and (**b**) critical landmarks

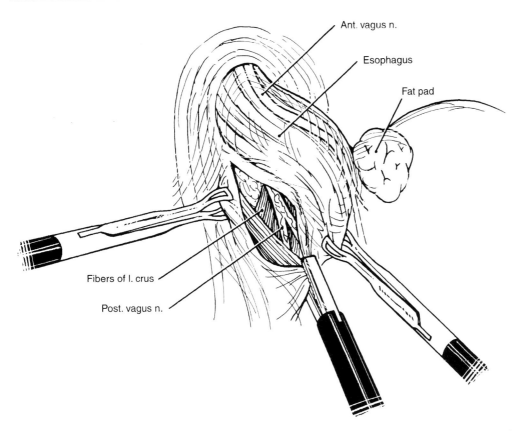

Fig. 5.5 Creation of a window below the left crus in Nissen fundoplication. Critical landmarks

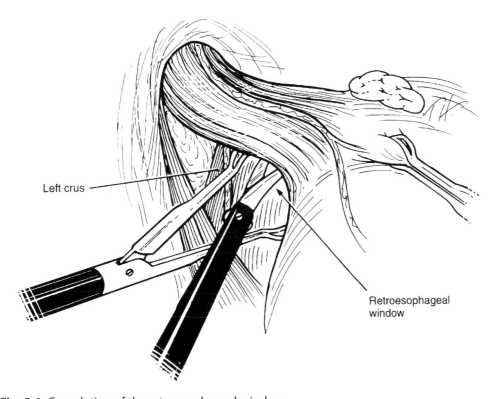

Fig. 5.6 Completion of the retroesophageal window

■ **Division of the Phrenoesophageal Membrane.** The phrenoesophageal membrane is divided after it has been dissected out from the anterior aspect of the esophagus, preserving the terminal branches of the anterior vagus nerve. This will expose the fat pad indicating the position of the angle of His and the gastroesophageal junction (Fig. 5.7). The dissection can be accomplished with harmonic shears.

At this point, a change in the angulation of the 30-degree laparoscope allows identification of the left crus on the left side of the esophagus. After this is done, the passage behind the esophagus can be completed. A right-angled dissector passed from the right to the left side will allow safe insertion of a Penrose drain around the esophagus; the drain is then clipped or endolooped to itself to prevent dislodgement from around the esophagus. This clear dissection technique avoids blind creation of the retroesophageal window, with the possibility of injury to the posterior aspect of the esophagus as reported in some series, leading to perforation and delayed mediastinitis. Once the Penrose drain is around the esophagus, it is pulled up and the window is enlarged by division of some avascular adhesions (Fig. 5.8a, b). In some patients, a small artery is found, which requires division between clips.

■ **Division of the Short Gastric Vessels.** Many surgeons are reluctant to perform this step because of the potential threat of bleeding. Nevertheless, it can be performed safely if simple rules are followed. The stomach is grabbed by the left grasper of the surgeon, and the lateral aspect of the gastrosplenic ligament is put under tension superiorly and

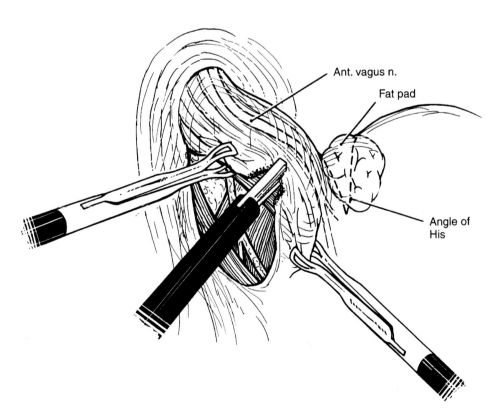

Fig. 5.7 Division of the phrenoesophageal membrane with preservation of both vagus nerves

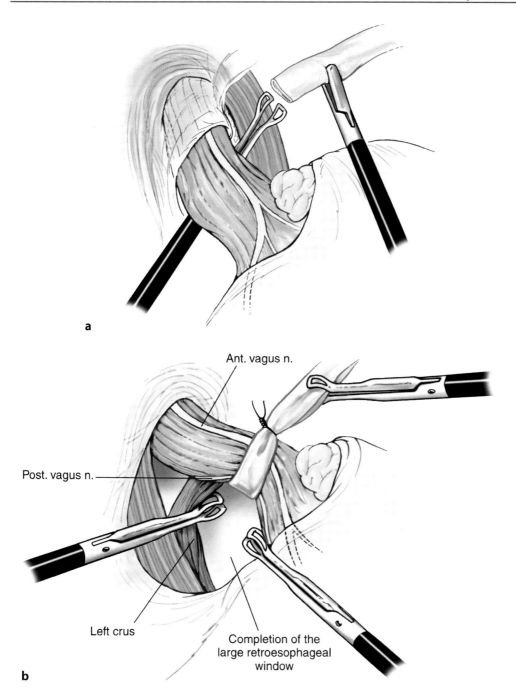

a

Ant. vagus n.

Post. vagus n.

Left crus

Completion of the
large retroesophageal
window

b

Fig. 5.8 (**a**) Insertion of a 12 cm Penrose drain around the esophagus, and (**b**) securing the drain with an Endoloop

laterally by the atraumatic grasper of the first assistant. An atraumatic grasper is important here to be able to control bleeding in the ligament (Fig. 5.9).

The surgeon then divides the short gastric vessels, starting at mid fundus and advancing superiorly until a point is reached where these vessels are very short and close to the spleen. The harmonic scalpel (Ethicon Endo Surgery, Inc.) is used in a scooping motion to create windows between the short gastric vessels (Fig. 5.10a). Some of the larger vessels are secured between clips (Fig. 5.10b).

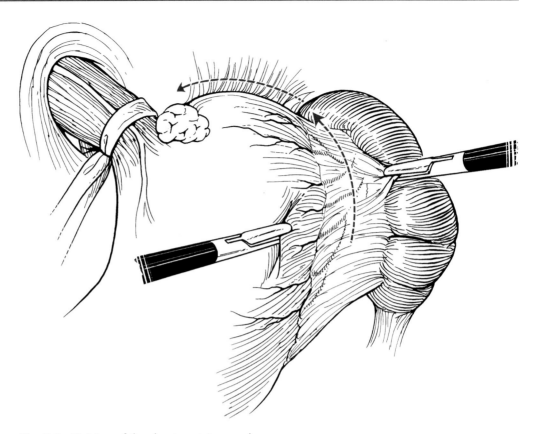

Fig. 5.9 Division of the short gastric vessels

The dissection proceeds superiorly until the final short gastric vessel is divided (Fig. 5.11). The last short gastric vessels are closely attached to the spleen, and should be divided cautiously using a right angle to carefully dissect each vessel. A useful trick is to move the scope to the most lateral left trocar to look at the posterior aspect of the stomach to ensure that no short gastric vessels adherent to the peri-pancreatic fat are missed. This complete division of all short gastric vessels and subsequent mobilization of the fundus allows for the creation of a very floppy wrap.

The dissection is complete upon rolling the mobilized fundus medially when one can see the left crus and the Penrose drain around the esophagus at the left side of the esophagus.

The next step is to identify the posterior aspect of the fundus and differentiate it from the anterior fundus. *In this procedure only the posterior fundus will be passed behind the esophagus.* This is the concept of a *balanced wrap.* To bring the posterior fundus around, one can push it gently into the retroesophageal window, or one can grab it with an atraumatic Babcock grasper.

The above procedure contrasts with the Rossetti operation in which a sling mechanism is created by passing the *anterior* aspect of the fundus around the esophagus and suturing it to another part (often the body) of the stomach. Unfortunately, this creates an unbalanced wrap, putting the gastroesophageal junction under lateral tension, twisting it, and potentially resulting in postoperative dysphagia (Fig. 5.12).

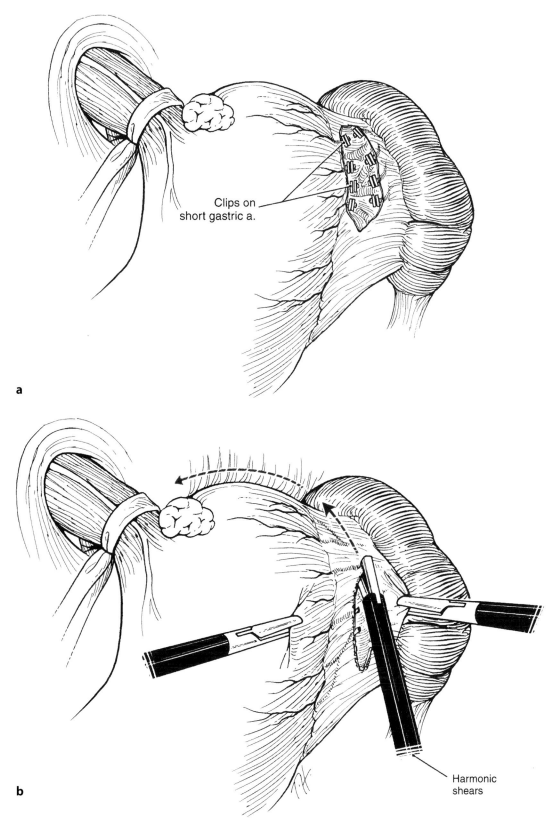

Clips on
short gastric a.

a

Harmonic
shears

b

Fig. 5.10 (**a**) Division of the gastrosplenic ligament using clips, and (**b**) division of the short
gastric vessels using harmonic scissors

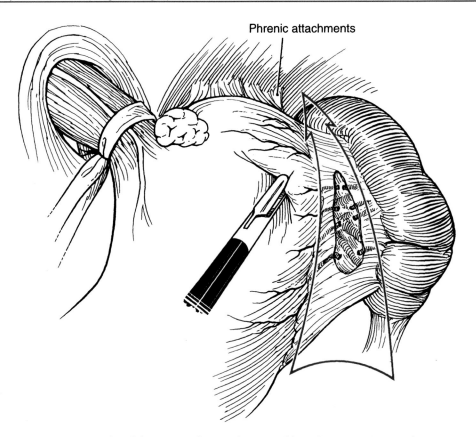

Fig. 5.11 Narrow angle of dissection during division of last short gastric vessels

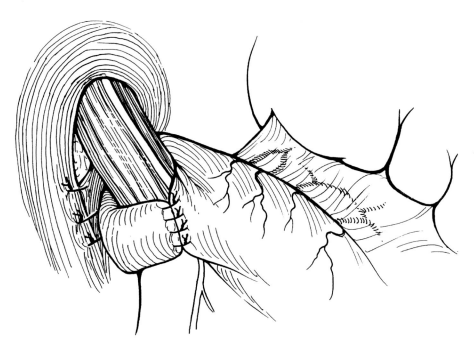

Fig. 5.12 Rosetti fundoplication (sling effect)

■ **Crural Closure and Fundoplication.** The crura are then closed behind the esophagus with three or four interrupted stitches of 2–0 Ethibond sutures on an SH needle point. The thread should be at least 35 in. (90 cm) if extracorporeal knotting is performed or six inches (15 cm) if intracorporeal knot tying is chosen (Fig. 5.13).

The knots are tied extracorporeally either by using a Roeder's knot-tying technique or by sliding each half knot using a knot pusher. Both techniques are acceptable and the surgeon should choose the one with which he or she is most comfortable. The closure is calibrated by passing a Babcock grasper between the esophagus and the last row of stitches to ensure that the closure is not too tight. After this, the wrap is passed through the retroesophageal window, with care being taken to pass the appropriate part of the posterior fundus as described above. One trick is to let the fundus lie behind the esophagus: if it stays in place, the wrap is probably not under tension; if it rolls back, another aspect of the fundus should be taken to ensure that the wrap is absolutely floppy.

The next step is insertion of a large (60 Fr) bougie by an experienced anesthesiologist under direct scrutiny by the surgeon. Cephalad esophageal retraction must be avoided in this process. Calibration around a large bougie leads to the creation of an appropriately floppy wrap that will allow efficient restoration of the resting pressure of the sphincter and good relaxation of the sphincter on swallowing. The wrap is sutured by placing two or three stitches of 2–0 Prolene on an SH needle (Fig. 5.14). The knots are tied appropriately, with six or seven throws being necessary. Care must be taken to pass the suture through the full thickness of the stomach, but only through muscle into the esophagus so as not to contaminate the gastroesophageal junction by a full-thickness bite into the esophageal mucosa. The wrap should have a maximum length of 2 cm.

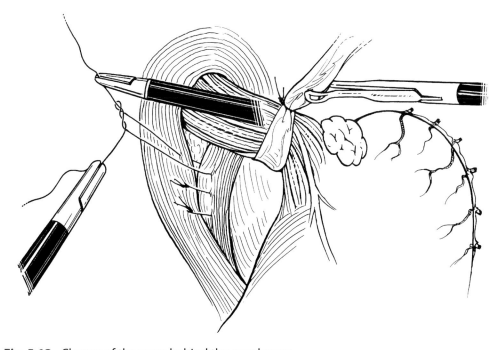

Fig. 5.13 Closure of the crura behind the esophagus

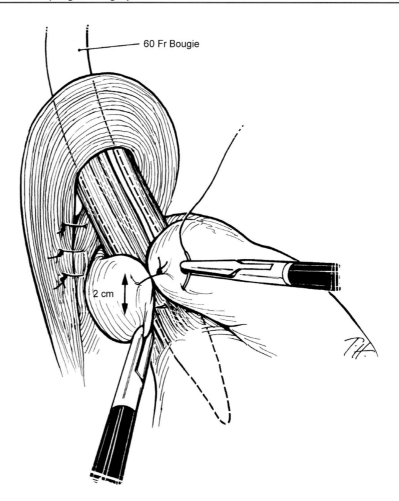

Fig. 5.14 Short floppy fundoplication around a 60Fr bougie

Finally, the hiatal area is irrigated and a careful check is done for hemostasis. All fluids must be aspirated with the patient in a normal position to avoid residual fluid in the left hypochondrium. The ports are removed and all wounds are closed. A nasogastric tube is left in place for 24 h selectively.

Postoperative Course

Patients are encouraged and assisted to ambulate the same night after surgery. They are started on a liquid diet on the first postoperative day and allowed a very soft diet later. A patient who has normal vital signs, urinates well, and tolerates fluids and a soft diet is authorized to leave the hospital as early as the first or second postoperative day.

Early in the author's experience, all patients were given a gastrographin upper gastrointestinal study to ensure the wrap was in place and there was no leak. This is no longer done as confidence in the operation has been gained. Patients are advised of the importance of continuing on a very soft diet for about 30 days, fractioning the meals to five a day and avoiding carbonated sodas, meat, chicken, and bread. This minimizes the temporary swallowing discomfort that some patients experience.

Management of Complications

During the operation one may encounter bleeding, esophageal perforation, or splenic injuries. Splenic injuries are more frequently reported in open surgery and have become rare incidents in laparoscopic procedures. Two other problems might be encountered postoperatively: mediastinitis and subphrenic abscesses due to delayed esophageal necrosis, mechanical problems associated with a tight wrap, a slipped wrap, or early breakdown of the repair.

■ **Bleeding During the Procedure.** Some bleeding may occur during the process of dissecting behind the esophagus while creating the window. It is very hazardous to use electrocautery to stop the bleeding, especially in the blind area behind the esophagus. Compression with a piece of laparoscopic 2 × 2 in. gauze inserted through one of the trocars will usually control a minor bleed, such as from a small esophageal vein.

More severe bleeding may occur during division of the short gastric vessels, with the formation of a large hematoma in the gastrosplenic ligament that renders the dissection very difficult. It is therefore advisable to control the vessel immediately using an atraumatic clamp, clean and irrigate around the area, and then selectively apply clips to the bleeding site. The flat blade of the harmonic shears also works well in this situation.

Bleeding from an injury to the spleen is more difficult to control. Again, compression using 2 × 2 in. gauze is best employed, together with application of high-voltage monopolar current. If the splenic injury is not very large it may be possible to control the situation by applying collagen pads or other hemostatic products, such as Tisseel. If the bleeding is not controllable, the decision for conversion should be made promptly.

■ **Perforation of the Esophagus.** Esophageal perforation can occur during insertion of the large bougie. Such an incident is *preventable* if the bougie is inserted very slowly by an experienced anesthesiologist under supervision of the surgeon, carefully avoiding anterior retraction of the esophagus that angles the esophagus and leads to perforation (Fig. 5.15). If theperforation is recognized during the operation, and if the level of skill of the surgeon is high, the perforation can be closed laparoscopically and the fundoplication can be applied as a "plasty" procedure to cover it. Otherwise, conversion should be the rule for repair.

Any postoperative fever, tachycardia, or signs of intraabdominal sepsis can indicate esophageal perforation. Even a modest left pleural effusion should raise the alarm. This complication is severe and may lead to death; it should be ruled out immediately by a gastrographin swallow or a CT scan with oral and IV contrast followed by upper gastrointestinal endoscopy if necessary. If an esophageal perforation is confirmed and the patient has become severely septic, the only option is to operate immediately to divert the esophagus. Diversion is the safest way to save the patient's life and is preferable to a primary closure of the perforation. At this stage, it is best done using an *open* approach.

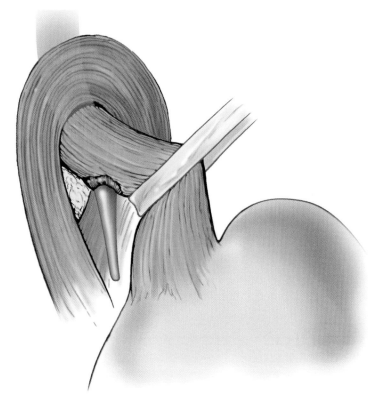

Fig. 5.15 A common site of esophageal perforation on its posterior aspect

■ **Mechanical Problems.** Mechanical problems can be related to a tight, slipped, or broken wrap (Fig. 5.16).

These complications are *avoidable* because they are the result of a flawed technique. *Breakdown of the wrap* is due to dislocation of the sutures from the stomach and the esophagus. *Tightness* is due to nondivision of the short gastric vessels or noncalibration with a 60 Fr bougie. Tightness leading to dysphagia is an indication for dilation via upper GI endoscopy. If this is not successful, then the wrap has to be taken down. This can be done laparoscopically if the surgeon has special expertise, but it is safer to perform the operation using an open approach. The same remark applies to breakdown of the repair due to improper suturing. One should also distinguish a *slipped wrap* caused by the sutures not involving the esophagus and allowing the stomach to "slip" behind the wrap from a wrap that was initially performed around the body of the stomach and not around the gastroesophageal junction; they present similarly on X-ray.

A final comment should be made about the *short esophagus*. This is usually defined on endoscopy as a distance of more than 4 cm between the gastroesophageal junction and the crura. A short esophagus is usually associated with a complication such as a stricture or Barrett's esophagus. Technically it is possible to lower the gastroesophageal junction by a careful dissection of the esophagus in the mediastinum. With a very short esophagus, the only possibility could be to approach it through a thoracotomy and perform a lengthening procedure (such as a Collis–Belsey). While it may be possible to bring the "short" esophagus down, it is definitely safer to perform an

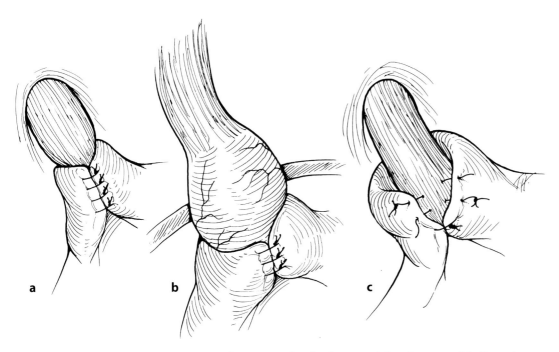

Fig. 5.16 Mechanical complications after Nissen fundoplication: (**a**) tight wrap; (**b**) slipped wrap; (**c**) breakdown of the repair

antireflux procedure through a thoracic approach than to struggle to put a wrap inappropriately under tension around the body of the stomach or around the esophageal body itself. An elegant solution is the performance of a laparoscopic abdominal Collis gastroplasty.

A 48 French bougie is inserted into the stomach and positioned along the lesser curvature, under laparoscopic control. A 21 or 25 size circular stapler is introduced through one of the left lateral ports, which is enlarged to accommodate a 33 mm port. The central rod of the stapler perforates first the posterior and then the anterior gastric wall at a distance of about 4 cm from the angle of His, and the anvil is introduced into the abdominal cavity. The anvil is connected to the rod using specially designed laparoscopic forceps. The circular stapler is fired, thus creating a punched hole in the stomach. An endolinear cutter 60 is then introduced and the jaws placed in the gastric hole with the tip pointing at the angle of His. The cutter is fired thus creating a Collis lengthening gastroplasty (Fig. 5.17). The staple lines are inspected and checked with methylene blue for potential leaks. Two running sutures will secure the staple lines. The procedure is completed with the creation of a floppy Nissen fundoplication with the remaining fundus.

Another technique is a fundectomy with a Collis–Nissen. After mobilizing the fundus, it is divided and resected using several firings of horitzontally placed cutters with blue loads. Then an articulating cutter, which has been calibrated with a 40 Fr Bougie, is placed vertically along the side of the esophagus and fired, creating a lengthened "neoesophagus." The fundus is then wrapped around this neoesophagus in the usual manner.

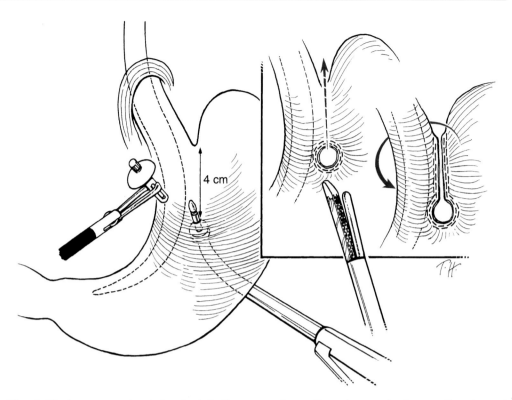

4 cm

Fig. 5.17 Laparoscopic abdominal Collis gastroplasty. *Dotted arrow* indicates direction of firing of the stapler. *Solid curved arrow* indicates fundoplication

Toupet Posterior Partial Fundoplication

The Toupet operation consists of a posterior partial wrap and is usually reserved for patients with poor esophageal motility on preoperative manometry, with a positive 24 pH study indicating gastroesophageal reflux disease. These patients benefit from a partial 270-degree wrap rather than a 360-degree wrap that puts the patient at risk of postoperative failure due to dysphagia.

The original Toupet fundoplication was an extensive procedure with mobilization of the preaortic fascia behind the posterior fundus, allowing sliding of the fundus in the retroesophageal window. The operation also fixed the wrap to the crura on each side. The right part of the posterior fundus was fixed to the right crura and the left part of the fundus was fixed to the left crura; then both aspects of the wrap were fixed to the anterior aspect of the esophagus, producing four lines of sutures of three sutures each, totaling 12 sutures. Two more stitches incorporated the esophagus, resulting in a wrap fixed with 14 sutures. The problem with the technique is that it transforms a mobile wrap into a wrap fixed to the crura (Fig. 5.18).

It is well known that with belching or vomiting, or simple swallowing, the gastroesophageal junction has vertical movements that put a wrap under tension. Moreover, the crura have closing and opening mechanisms on respiration that increases tension in the wrap with the risk of breakdown of the repair with time.

An elegant solution is presented by the Fekete–Toupet modified fundoplication (Fig. 5.19). *This consists of closure of the crura* behind the esophagus and passage of the posterior fundus behind the esophagus, as with the Nissen fundoplication described

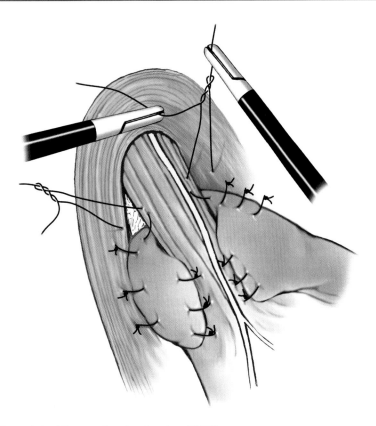

Fig. 5.18 The original Toupet fundoplication (270°)

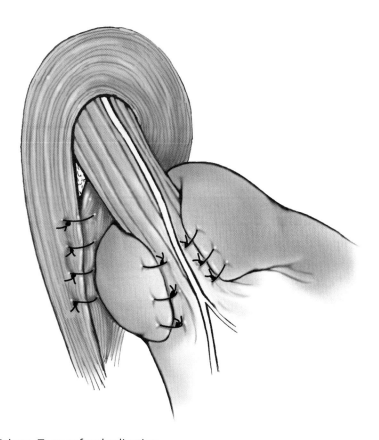

Fig. 5.19 Modified Fekete–Toupet fundoplication

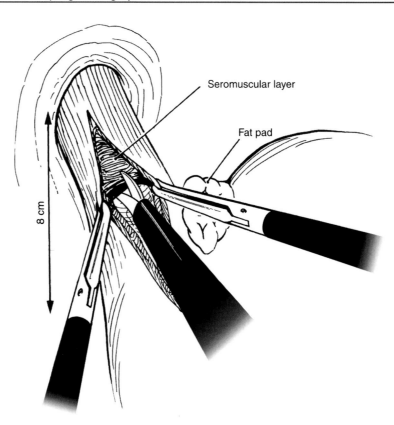

Fig. 5.22 Esophageal Heller myotomy using the scissors

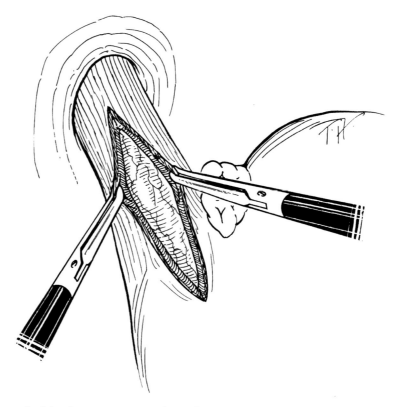

Fig. 5.23 End of the dissection in esophageal myotomy

The patient position is the same as for Nissen fundoplication. The port positions are also the same.

On starting the esophageal myotomy it is essential to visualize the gastroesophageal junction. This is achieved by division of the phrenoesophageal membrane, the dissection proceeding from right to left. The fat pad indicates the angle of His. At this point the gastroesophageal junction is revealed.

The myotomy is started on the esophagus itself, and should be about 8 cm long. The inferior aspect of the myotomy should be started just at the junction between the esophagus and the stomach, and extend 10–20 mm on the gastric side. First, two graspers are used to grasp the esophagus. A scissor is employed for the myotomy after creating a small groove in the muscular layer of the esophagus to allow its introduction (Fig. 5.22). By combining a spreading motion between the two layers of the esophagus, and dissection with the scissor just dividing the muscular layer, it is possible to see the white, pale esophageal mucosa bulging between the layers (Fig. 5.23). Traction on the layers, with electrocautery by the hook, will allow safe division of the final muscular layers of the diseased esophageal segment.

On completion of the myotomy, the integrity of the mucosa is tested by filling the esophagus with about 300 mL of diluted methylene blue. If a small mucosal perforation is revealed, it is possible to insert a stitch of 3–0 Prolene suture, but it is advisable to add an anterior fundoplication (Dor) to the myotomy as an extra safety measure, and to prevent reflux postoperatively.

Finally, if one believes that measures are needed to prevent postoperative gastroesophageal reflux, it is also possible to add a posterior 180–270-degree Toupet fundoplication.

Esophageal Myotomy for Achalasia

Bilateral Truncal Vagotomy

Vagotomies

Truncal vagotomy is not a difficult procedure and should take no more than about 20 min. The patient setup and the surgeon's position between the patient's legs, with the assistants on each side, are the same as for all approaches to the hiatus. The landmarks are also the same: the avascular aspect of the lesser sac that, once opened, leads to the caudate lobe of the liver, and the right crus of the diaphragm at the left side of the caudate lobe (Fig. 5.24a).

The right crus of the diaphragm is grasped by the left grasper in the left hand of the surgeon, and the harmonic shears are used to create a small space between the esophagus and the right crus. This space is avascular. With spreading movements of both the shears and the grasper, the space is enlarged, leading to visualization of the left crus of the diaphragm. If the left crus is not immediately recognized, it is possible to follow the right crus down until it connects with the left crus.

The search for the right vagus nerve begins at this point. It usually lies on the back wall of the esophagus, or next to either the right or left crus. The posterior vagus nerve is a big trunk that cannot be missed: it is white, with small veins running on its surface, and it is elastic and resistant to pulling. The posterior vagus is divided between clips, and a piece is sent for pathological examination (Fig. 5.24b).

At this point it is possible to divide the phrenoesophageal membrane that covers most of the branches of the left vagus nerve. The left grasper is used to pull up on the membrane,

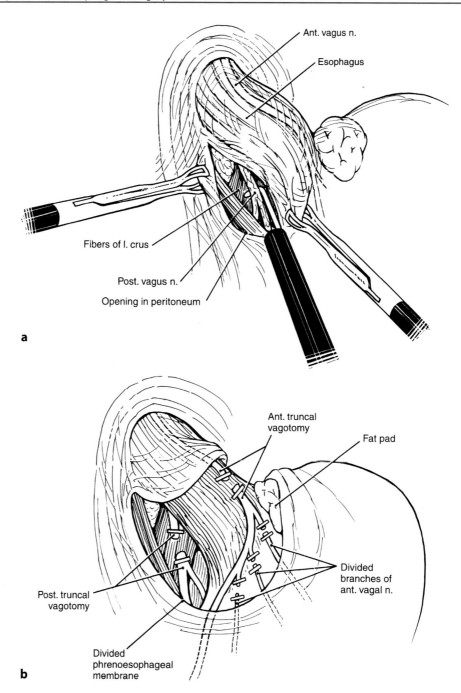

Fig. 5.24 Bilateral truncal vagotomy: (**a**) landmarks, and (**b**) divisions of vagus nerves

while the harmonic shears create a dissection plane between the esophagus and the membrane. Clips can be placed as the esophageal membrane is divided to avoid any oozing of blood, or the harmonic shears can be used. Dissection is continued until the angle of His is reached in the area of the fat pad. It should now be possible to recognize one or two trunks of the left vagus nerve, which will be divided in the same manner as the right vagus nerve.

A 30-degree laparoscope should be used to check the posterior aspect of the left border of the esophagus. In this area one should look in particular for the "criminal" nerve branches of Grassi that usually run on the left side of the esophagus. It is crucial to

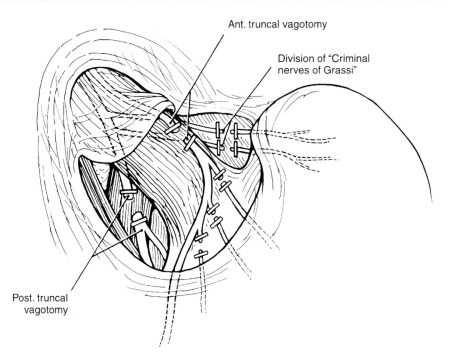

Ant. truncal vagotomy

Division of "Criminal nerves of Grassi"

Post. truncal vagotomy

Fig. 5.25 Division of the "criminal" nerve branches of Grassi in bilateral truncal vagotomy

divide these to ensure a total vagotomy (Fig. 5.25). If they are missed, the chances of recurrence of an ulcer are greatly increased. If necessary, one should go back and create a small window behind the esophagus to enable division of these "criminal" branches.

Finally, the area is thoroughly rinsed and aspirated, and hemostasis completed as needed.

Highly Selective Vagotomy

This operation proceeds in the same manner as for open surgery. It is important to recognize the landmarks that are part of the operation: the greater gastric nerves of Latarjet, terminal branches of the right and left trunks of vagus nerves, and the crow's foot at the antrum. Each crow's foot has between three and five branches. The greater nerves of Latarjet before their ending give rise to several fundic branches that need to be divided to assure a complete highly selective vagotomy (Fig. 5.26).

The beginning of the operation is tedious because one has to create a dissection space in a very narrow angle. This is achieved by dividing a large vessel next to the last branch of the crow's foot, which will permit division of all the branches together with the vessels, starting from below and moving in a cephalad direction towards the esophagus. It is important to stay close to the lesser curvature of the stomach and avoid the main trunk of the gastric nerve. Indeed, a hematoma may cause compression of the nerve, or even incorrect identification of the nerve and the risk of injury will be greater.

The technique of dissection is to create a window between each vessel and nerve. These windows are created with harmonic shears. Then with a scooping motion each vessel is mobilized and clips are applied (Fig. 5.27). It is important to start with each leaf, of which there are usually three:

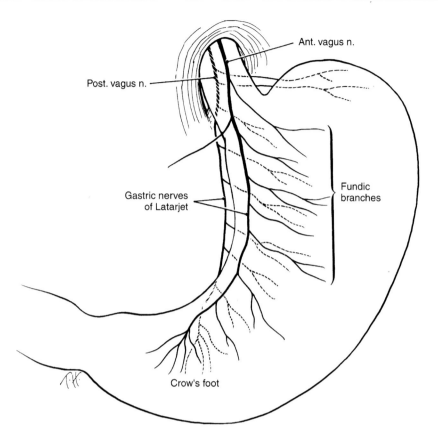

Fig. 5.26 Anatomical landmarks in highly selective vagotomy

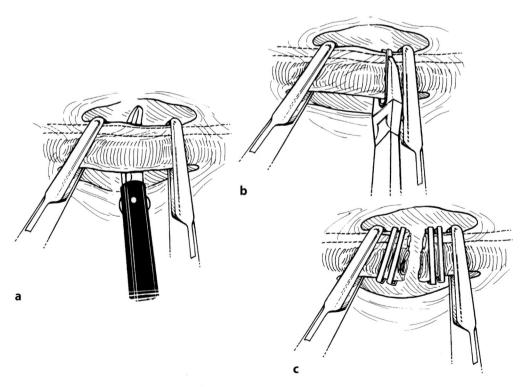

Fig. 5.27 The general technique of division of vessels, applying to highly selective vagotomy, gastrectomy, splenectomy, and Nissen fundoplication. (**a**) dissection with curved scissors, (**b**) placement of clips, (**c**) division of vessels between double clips

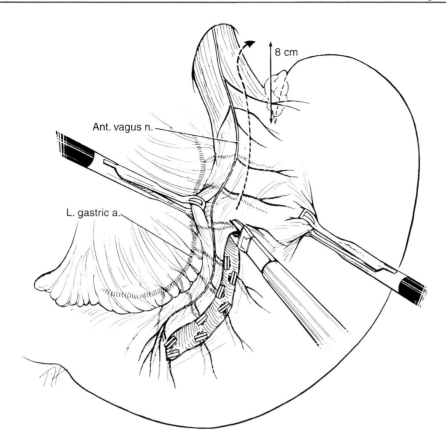

Fig. 5.28 Highly selective vagotomy using clips

- An anterior leaf containing all the vessels and nerve branches of the anterior greater nerve of Latarjet
- A middle leaf, usually devoid of any vessels
- A posterior leaf containing vessels and the branches of the posterior greater nerve of Latarjet

It is imperative to go all the way up to the gastroesophageal junction, and then as in open surgery to continue on the anterior aspect of the esophagus until the angle of His is reached. Then division is started again at the antrum and proceeds in a cephalad manner until the lesser sac is completely opened, which will signify division of all the fundic branches of the two greater nerves of Laterjet. It is important to make sure that at least 3 in. (8 cm) of the esophagus is skeletonized superiorly, but care must be taken not to divide or injure the main trunk of the vagus nerves themselves (Fig. 5.28).

If there is bleeding of a small vessel next to the lesser curvature it is possible to grab the vessel. However, sometimes it is as convenient and more effective to grab the lesser curvature itself with an atraumatic clamp, which should always be available when performing this operation. Subsequently, the general principles apply: pan out the video camera, irrigate and clean the area around the bleeding, and then do selective hemostasis by using either clips or electrocautery.

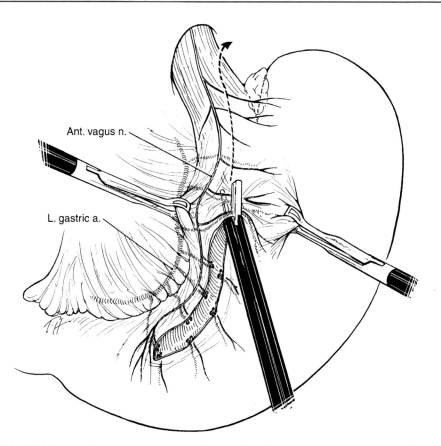

Ant. vagus n.

L. gastric a.

Fig. 5.29 Highly selective vagotomy using harmonic scissors

Caution is necessary when using extensive electrocautery next to the lesser curvature, which could lead to injury to the organ and a seromuscular perforation. The author therefore recommends the use of clips rather than monopolar electrocautery on the lesser curvature itself. Alternatively, a highly selective vagotomy can be performed using harmonic scissors (Fig. 5.29). The great advantage is that there is no need to create windows. Harmonic scissors are welding tools that enable one to perform the operation safely in less than 2 h, minimizing lateral injury to the stomach or to the nerves of Latarjet.

Lesser Curvature Seromyotomy and Posterior Truncal Vagotomy

This is a technique that has been popularized in open surgery by T. V. Taylor and was performed by the author as the first published laparoscopic vagotomy technique. It combines a posterior truncal vagotomy, as described earlier, with an anterior lesser curvature seromyotomy. The anterior lesser curvature seromyotomy starts at the posterior aspect of the angle of His, proceeds parallel 10–15 mm from the lesser curvature, and ends approximately 6 cm from the pylorus at the first branch of the crow's foot.

Both aspects of the stomach are grasped and the dissection is started by creating a small groove between the graspers, using an electrical hook. The combination of traction by the graspers and the electrocautery leads to exposure of the submucosal layer, which can be recognized by its blue color. It is *not* necessary to go beyond the submucosal layer.

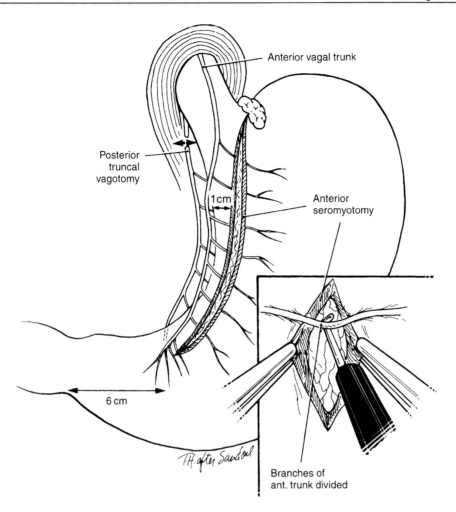

Anterior vagal trunk

Posterior
truncal
vagotomy

1 cm

Anterior
seromyotomy

6 cm

T.H. after Sandoz

Branches of
ant. trunk divided

Fig. 5.30 Posterior truncal vagotomy and anterior lesser curvature seromyotomy

If one crosses this layer, oozing will be encountered. The risk of opening the mucosa at this point is great. If one stays at the submucosal layer, the risk of opening the mucosa is absolutely minimal.

Starting at the angle of His, the seromyotomy goes down to include the last branch of the crow's foot. It is recommended that two or three large vessels running on the anterior aspect of the stomach are divided before one starts the seromyotomy, as initially advocated by Taylor in open surgery (Fig. 5.30). This is done by using the harmonic shears.

When the seromyotomy is complete, a continuous suture is placed in an overlap fashion to bring the two edges of the stomach on each other. This will prevent nerve regeneration and blood oozing, and therefore postoperative adhesions (Fig. 5.31).

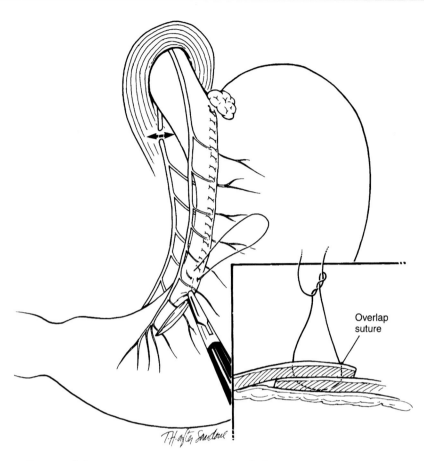

Overlap
suture

Fig. 5.31 Closure of the seromyotomy in an overlap fashion

Alexander HC, Hendler RS (1996) Laparoscopic reoperation on failed antireflux procedures: report of two patients. Surg Laparosc Endosc 6(2):147–149

Anvari M, Allen C, Borm A (1995) Laparoscopic Nissen fundoplication is a satisfactory alternative to long-term omeprazole therapy. Br J Surg 82(7):938–942

Anvari M, Allen C, Moran LA (1996) Immediate and delayed effects of laparoscopic Nissen fundbplication on pulmonary function. Surg Endosc 10(12):1171–1175

Awad W, Csendes A, Braghetto I et al (1997) Laparoscopic highly selective vagotomy: technical considerations and preliminary results in 119 patients with duodenal ulcer or gastroesophageal reflux disease. World J Surg 21(3):261–268

Aye RW, Hill LD, Kraemer SJ, Snopkowski P (1994) Early results with the laparoscopic Hill repair. Am J Surg 167(5):542–546

Bell RCW, Hanna P, Powers B, Sabel J, Hruza D (1996) Clinical and manometric results of laparoscopic partial (Toupet) and complete (Rosetti—Nissen) fundoplication. Surg Endosc 10(7):724–728

Branicki FJ, Nathanson LK (1994a) Minimal access gastroduodenal surgery. Aust NZ J Surg 64(9):589–598

Branicki FJ, Nathanson LK (1994b) Minimal access gastroduodenal surgery. Aust NZ J Surg 64(9):589–598

Bittner HB, Meyers WC, Brazer SR, Pappas TN (1994) Laparoscopic Nissen fundoplication: operative results and short-term follow-up. Am J Surg 167(1):193–198

Brody FJ, Trad KS (1997) Comparison of acid reduction in antiulcer operations. Surg Endosc 11(2):123–125

Broeders JA, Rijnhart-de Jong HG, Draaisma WA, Bredenoord AJ, Smout AJ, Gooszen HG (2009) Ten-year outcome of laparoscopic and conventional nissen fundoplication: randomized clinical trial. Ann Surg 250(5):698–706

Cadiere GB, Flimpens I, Bruyns J (1994a) Laparoscopic proximal gastric vagotomy. Endosc Surg Allied Technol 2(2):105–108

Cadiere GB, Houben JJ, Bruyns J, Himpens J, Panzer JM, Gelin M (1994b) Laparoscopic Nissen fundoplication: technique and preliminary results. Br J Surg 81(3):400–403

Cadiere GB, Himpens I, Bruyns I (1995) How to avoid esophageal perforation while performing laparoscopic dissection of the hiatus. Surg Endosc 9(4):450–452

Campos GM, Vittinghoff E, Rabl C, Takata M, Gadenstätter M, Lin F, Ciovica R (2009) Endoscopic and surgical treatments for achalasia: a systematic review and meta-analysis. Ann Surg 249(1):45–57

Casas AT, Gadacz TR (1996) Laparoscopic management of pepti ulcer disease. Surg Clin N Am 76(3):515–522

Collard JM, de Gheldere CA, De Kock M, Otte JB, Kestens PI (1994) Laparoscopic antireflux surgery. What is real progress? Ann Surg 220(2):146–154

Collet D, Cadiere GB (1995) Conversions and complications of laparoscopic treatment of gastroesophageal reflux disease. Formation for the development of laparoscopic surgery for gastroesophageal reflux. Disease Group. Am J Surg 169(6):622–626

Croce E, Azzola M, Golia M et al (1994) Laparoscopic posterior truncal vagotomy and anterior proximal gastric vagotomy. Endosc Surg Allied Technol 2(2):113–116

Csendes A (2007) Prosthetic hiatal closure during laparoscopic Nissen fundoplication. Arch Surg 142(11):1110–1111

Dallemagne B, Weerts JM, Jahaes C et al (1991) Laparoscopic Nissen fundoplication: preliminary report. Surg Laparosc Endosc 1:138–141

Dallemagne B, Weerts JM, Jehaes C, Markiewicz S, Lombard R (1994) Laparoscopic highly selective vagotomy. Br J Surg 81(4):554–556

Dallemagne B, Weerts JM, Jehaes C, Markiewicz S (1996) Causes of failure of laparoscopic antirefiux operations. Surg Endosc 10(3):305–310

De Meester TR, Bonavina L, Albertucci M (1986) Nissen fundoplication for gastroesophageal reflux disease: evaluation of primary repair in 100 consecutive patients. Ann Surg 204:9–20

DePaula AL, Hashiba K, Bafutto M, Machado CA (1995) Laparoscopic reoperations after failed and complicated antireflux operations. Surg Endosc 9(6):681–686

Donahue PE, Griffith C, Richter HM (1996) A 50-year perspective upon selective gastric vagotomy. Am J Surg 172(1):9–12

Dor J, Humbert P, Dor V et al (1962) L'interêt de la technique de Nissen modifiée dans la prevention du reflux après cardiomyotomie extramuqueuse de Heller. Mem Acad Chir 88:877–884

Dubois F (1994) Vagotomies—laparoscopic or thoracoscopic approach. Endosc Surg Allied Technol 2(2):100–104

Ferguson CM, Rattner DW (1995) Initial experience with laparoscopic Nissen fundoplication. Am Surg 61(1):21–23

Fletcher DR (1997) Peptic disease: can we afford current management? Aust NZ Surg 67(2–3):75–80

Fontaumard E, Espalieu P, Boulez J (1995) Laparoscopic Nissen—Rossetti fundoplication. First results. Surg Endosc 9(8):869–873

Gee DW, Andreoli MT, Rattner DW (2008) Measuring the effectiveness of laparoscopic antireflux surgery: long-term results. Arch Surg 143(5):482–487

Geagea T (1991) Laparoscopic Nissen fundoplication: preliminary report on the cases. Surg Endosc 5:1170–1173

Gotley DC, Smithers BM, Rhodes M (1996) Laparoscopic surgery for duodenal ulcer: first results of a multicentre study applying a personal procedure. Br J Surg 83(4):547–550

Hallerback B, Glise H, Johansson B, Radmark T (1994) Laparoscopic Rosetti fundoplication. Surg Endosc 8(12):1417–1422

Hayes N, Raimes SA, Griffin SM (1994) Laparoscopic vagotomy: an operation for the 1990s? Ann R Coil Surg Eng 76(3):211

Helling TS (1995) Perforation of the stomach during laparoscopic Nissen fundoplication in a patient on chronic corticosteroid therapy. Surg Endosc 9(10):1146

Heloury Y, Plattner V, Mirallie E, Gerard P, Lejus C (1996) Laparoscopic Nissen fundoplication with simultaneous percutaneous endoscopic gastrostomy in children. Surg Endosc 10(8):837–841

Hinder RA, Filipi CJ, Wetscher G, Neary P, DeMeester TR, Perdikis G (1994) Laparoscopic Nissen fundoplication is an effective treatment for gastroesophageal reflux disease. Ann Surg 220(4):472–481

Hinder RA, Raiser F, Katkhouda N, McBride PJ, Perdikis G, Lund RJ (1995) Results of Nissen fundoplication. A cost analysis. Surg Endosc 9(12):1328–1332

Hunter JG, Swanstrom L, Waring JP (1996a) Dysphagia after laparoscopic antireflux surgery. The impact of operative technique. Ann Surg 224(1):51–57

Hunter JG, Trus TL, Branum GD, Waring JP, Wood WC (1996b) A physiologic approach to laparoscopic fundoplication for gastroesophageal reflux disease. Ann Surg 223(6):673–685

Incarbone R, Peters JH, Heimbucher J, Dvorak D, Bremner CG, DeMeester TR (1995) A contemporaneous comparison of hospital charges for laparoscopic and open Nissen fundoplication. Surg Endosc 9(2):151–154

Jamieson GG, Watson DI, Britten-Jones R, Mitchell PC, Anvari M (1994) Laparoscopic Nissen fundoplication. Ann Surg 220(2):137–145

Jobe BA, Kim CY, Minjarez RC, O'Rourke R, Chang EY, Hunter JG (2006) Simplifying minimally invasive transhiatal esophagectomy with the inversion approach: Lessons learned from the first 20 cases. Arch Surg 141(9):857–865

Johnson AG (1994) Management of peptic ulcer. Br J Surg 81(2):161–163

Katkhouda N, Steichen F, Ravitch M, Welter R, Mouiel J (1989) Integrated anastomotic resection in esogastric surgery. Lyon Chir 85:190–191

Katkhouda N, Khalil M, Grant S, Manhas S, Velmahos G, Umbach T, Kaiser A (2002) Andre Toupet: surgeon technician par excellence. Ann Surg 235:591–599

Kauer WK, Peters JH, DeMeester TR, Heimbucher J, Ireland AP, Bremner CG (1995) A tailored approach to antireflux surgery. J Ther Cardiovasc Surg 110(1):141–146

Khajanchee YS, Kanneganti S, Leatherwood AE, Hansen PD, Swanström LL (2005) Laparoscopic Heller myotomy with Toupet fundoplication: outcomes predictors in 121 consecutive patients. Arch Surg 140(9):827–833

Kilic A, Schuchert MJ, Pennathur A, Gilbert S, Landreneau RJ, Luketich JD (2009) Long-term outcomes of laparoscopic Heller myotomy for achalasia. Surgery 146(4): 826–831

Kollmorgen CF, Gunes S, Donohue JH, Thompson GB, Sarr MG (1996) Proximal gastric vagotomy. Comparison between open and laparoscopic methods in the canine model. Ann Surg 224(1):43–50

Laycock WS, Oddsdottir M, Franco A, Mansour K, Hunter JG (1995) Laparoscopic Nissen fundoplication is less expensive than open Belsey Mark IV. Surg Endosc 9(4):426–429

Laycock WS, Trus TL, Hunter IG (1996) New technology for the division of short gastric vessels during laparoscopic Nissen fundoplication. A prospective randomized trial. Surg Endosc 10(1):71–73

Lloyd DM, Robertson GS, Johnstone JM (1995) Laparoscopic Nissen fundoplication in children. Surg Endosc 9(7):781–785

McKernan JB (1994) Toupet partial fundoplication versus Nissen fundoplication. Laparoscopic repair of gastroesophageal reflux disease. Surg Endosc 8(8):851–856

Meehan JJ, Georgeson KB (1996) Laparoscopic fundoplication in infants and children. Surg Endosc 10(12):1154–1157

Menzies B, Branicki FJ, Nathanson L (1996) Laparoscopic Nissen fundoplication—200 consecutive cases. Gut 38(4):487–491

Mouiel J, Katkhouda N, Gugenheim J, Fabian P, Crafa F, Iovine L (1992) Endolaparoscopic Vagotomy. Chir Gastroenterologie 8:387–394 (in German)

Nguyen NT, Hinojosa MW, Smith BR, Chang KJ, Gray J, Hoyt D (2008) Minimally invasive esophagectomy: lessons learned from 104 operations. Ann Surg 248(6):1081–1091

Nissen R (1956) Eine Einfache operation zur beeinflussung der Refluxesophagitis. Schweitz Med Wochenschr 86:590–592

Naunheim KS, Landreneau RJ, Andrus CH, Ferson PF, Zachary PB, Keenan RI (1996) Laparoscopic fundoplication: a natural extension for the thoracic surgeon. Ann Thorac Surg 61(4):1062–1065

Ozmen V, Musleumanoglu M, Igci A, Bugra D (1995) Laparoscopic treatment of duodenal ulcer by bilateral truncal vagotomy and endoscopic balloon dilatation. J Laparoendosc Surg 5(1):21–26

Perry KA, Enestvedt CK, Pham T, Welker M, Jobe BA, Hunter JG, Sheppard BC (2009) Comparison of laparoscopic inversion esophagectomy and open transhiatal esophagectomy for high-grade dysplasia and stage I esophageal adenocarcinoma. Arch Surg 144(7):679–684

Peters JH, DeMeester TR (1996) Indications, benefits and outcome of laparoscopic Nissen fundoplication. Dig Dis 14(3):169–179

Peters JH, Heimbucher J, Kauer WK, Incarbone R, Bremner CG, DeMeester TR (1995) Clinical and physiologic comparison of laparoscopic and open Nissen fundoplication. J Am Coll Surg 180(4):385–393

Pitcher DE, Curet MJ, Martin DT et al (1994) Successful management of severe gastroesophageal reflux disease with laparoscopic Nissen fundoplication. Am J Surg 168(6): 547–553

Rantanen TK, Oksala NK, Oksala AK, Salo JA, Sihvo EI (2008) Complications in antireflux surgery: national-based analysis of laparoscopic and open fundoplications. Arch Surg 143(4):359–366

Rattner DW, Brooks DC (1995) Patient satisfaction following laparoscopic and open anti-reflux surgery. Arch Surg 130(3):289–293

Rebecchi F, Giaccone C, Farinella E, Campaci R, Morino M (2008) Randomized controlled trial of laparoscopic Heller myotomy plus Dor fundoplication versus Nissen fundoplication for achalasia: long-term results. Ann Surg 248(6):1023–1030

Rossetti M, Hall K (1977) Fundoplication in the treatment of gastroesophageal reflux in hiatal hernia. World J Surg 1:439–444

Sakuramachi S, Kimura T, Harada Y (1994) Experimental study of laparoscopic selective proximal vagotomy using a carbon dioxide laser. Surg Endosc 8(8):857–861

Scheepers JJ, Veenhof AA, van der Peet DL, van Groeningen C, Mulder C, Meijer S, Cuesta MA (2008) Laparoscopic transhiatal resection for malignancies of the distal esophagus: outcome of the first 50 resected patients. Surgery 143(2):278–285

Gastric Surgery 6

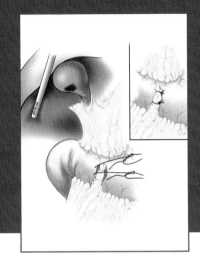

Pyloroplasty

A laparoscopic Heineke–Mikulicz pyloroplasty is performed in the same way as an open surgery. The most commonly encountered difficulty is recognition of the pyloric muscle through the scope.

For this reason it is advisable to note some of the landmarks that can be sought out, such as the pyloric vein of Mayo running on the muscle's surface and the change in diameter between the distal end of the stomach, the pyloric area, and the postpyloric region. It is usually possible to identify the pylorus using these anatomical features; however, in case of difficulty, the procedure can begin and once underway, a laparoscope can be inserted into the duodenum from the gastric side of the pyloroplasty, permitting recognition of the pyloric muscle by the change in caliber. Even then it can sometimes be difficult to identify the pylorus. In such cases, one can remove one trocar, insert a finger into the opening after partially deflating the abdomen and locate the pylorus by palpation (Fig. 6.1).

When the pyloroplasty has been created longitudinally, it is possible to suture it transversely exactly as in open surgery using interrupted stitches of 3–0 Prolene (the 4–0 suture used in open surgery is a little too thin and the risk of breaking the suture is greater). The 3–0 suture will give adequate strength for intracorporeal or extracorporal knot-tying; both are possible. The author advises buttressing the pyloroplasty with a small omental patch *as an extra safety measure* (Fig. 6.2).

N. Katkhouda, *Advanced Laparoscopic Surgery*,
DOI: 10.1007/978-3-540-74843-4_6, © Springer-Verlag Berlin Heidelberg 2011

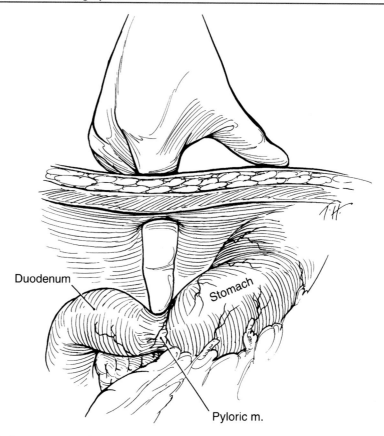

Fig. 6.1 A finger inserted in one of the port openings to palpate the pyloric muscle ("fingeroscopy")

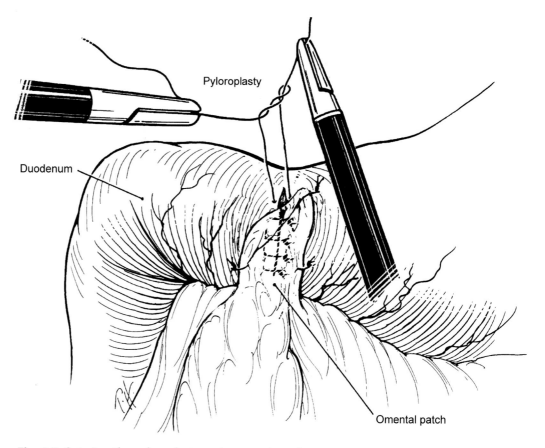

Fig. 6.2 Suturing the pyloroplasty and omental patch

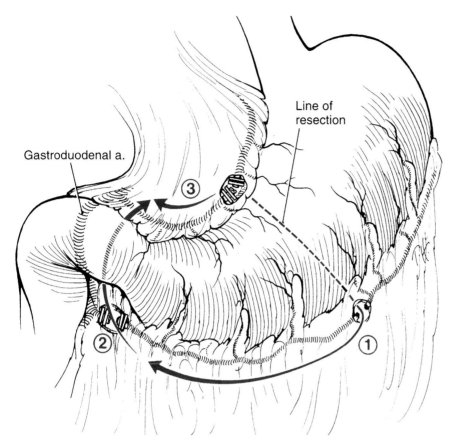

Fig. 6.3 Steps in laparoscopic gastrectomy

The technique for hemigastrectomy is the same as for antrectomy or distal gastrectomy.

An antrectomy can be combined with a bilateral truncal vagotomy in the treatment of gastric outlet obstruction. Technically the procedure is the same as for open surgery. The various steps are as follows (Fig. 6.3):

Vagotomy with Antrectomy or any Distal Gastrectomy

- Mobilization of the stomach's greater curvature by opening the gastrocolic ligament
- Dissection around the duodenum
- Division of the lesser omentum and the right gastric artery
- Transection of the duodenum
- Reconstruction by a Biliroth II gastrojejunostomy

Port Placement

Port placement is slightly different from other upper GI operations. The laparoscope should be able to conveniently access both the hiatus, in the case of a bilateral truncal vagotomy, and the greater curvature of the stomach, especially if the stomach is distended as in gastric outlet obstruction. It should therefore be inserted at the umbilicus. Placement for this and the remaining ports are depicted in Fig. 6.4. Before starting the operation it is important to insert a nasogastric tube to decompress the stomach, thus avoiding any injury to the stomach upon insertion of the Veress needle.

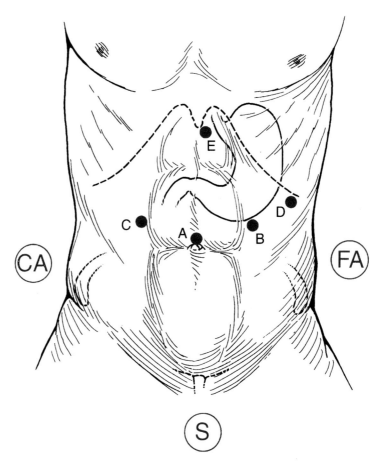

Fig. 6.4 Port positions for laparoscopic gastrectomy. *A* umbilicus; *B* surgeon's right hand (scissors); *C* surgeon's left hand (grasper), *D* assistant's grasper; *E* subxiphoid port. *S* surgeon; *FA* first assistant; *CA* camera assistant

Technique

The assistant begins the procedure by retracting the greater curvature of the stomach using a lateral port. The surgeon uses both hands to create windows in the gastrocolic ligament. It is advisable to start outside the gastroepiploic arcade and divide the arcade at the end of the dissection (Fig. 6.5).

A key maneuver to facilitate the operation is to change the position of the camera at each step of the procedure to obtain a more direct view of the structures involved with each phase of dissection. During the first step, while working on the gastrocolic ligament, the camera is placed at the umbilicus and the two hands of the surgeon are positioned on each side of the camera. As the dissection proceeds towards the antrum and the inferior aspect of the duodenum, the camera is moved to the port at the surgeon's right hand, and the two other ports are triangulated with the camera. These concepts are extremely important: (a) flexibility and mobility of the camera position, and (b) triangulation (Fig. 6.6).

Before the actual dissection is begun, it is important to check on the various landmarks: the curvatures of the stomach, the gastrocolic ligament and the gastroepiploic arcade, the inferior aspect of the antrum, the duodenum and the pyloric muscle, the lesser sac, and the right gastric artery. *The limit of the antrum and proposed site of the gastrojejunostomy is marked using electrocautery.*

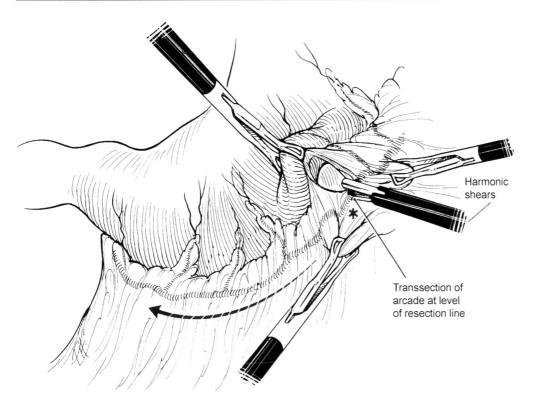

Fig. 6.5 Initiation of the gastrectomy. An *asterisk* marks the beginning of the dissection (division of the gastroepiploic arcade)

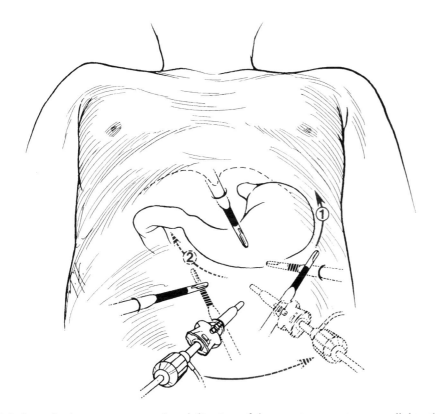

Fig. 6.6 Steps in the gastrectomy: *1* mobilization of the greater curvature parallel to the gastroepiploic arcade; *2* dissection of the antrum and inferior aspect of the duodenum

The dissection begins outside the gastroepiploic arcade using a harmonic scalpel. Transection of the right gastroepipoic artery is performed later. Few vessels are encountered, but one should stay very close to the gastroepiploic arcade to avoid injury of the transverse colon. Clips can be used for further hemostasis. Dissection proceeds slowly to the inferior aspect of the duodenum at the area where the proposed transection will be performed. At this point the right gastroepiploic artery is divided between clips, rather than applying electrocautery or using the harmonic shears alone.

■ **Division of the Right Gastroepiploic Artery and Retroduodenal Dissection.** Division of the right gastroepiploic artery precedes the posterior dissection of the duodenum. Using a right-angled dissector, exactly as it is used for dissection of the esophagus, a retroduodenal passage is created starting at the inferior aspect of the duodenum. Dissection then proceeds to the superior aspect of the duodenum and the right gastric artery is ligated between clips and divided. At this point a right-angled 10 mm dissector is introduced into the subxyphoid port to complete the dissection behind the duodenum, as the subxyphoid port is immediately in line with this dissection (Fig. 6.7).

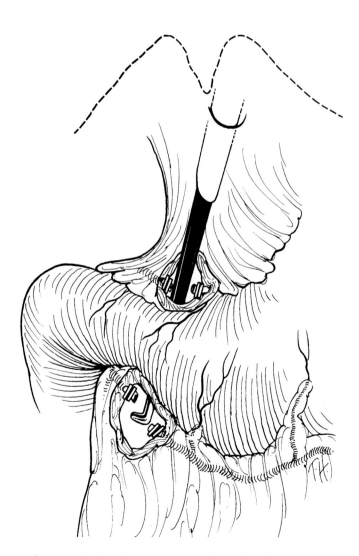

Fig. 6.7 Creation of a retroduodenal passage using the subxyphoid port

When the retroduodenal space has been created, an umbilical tape is passed around the duodenum and the window is enlarged. This permits the introduction of a 60 mm linear cutter through the same subxyphoid port in the same direction, and transection of the duodenum is carried out. Blue loads are typically used, but green loads are preferred if the duodenum is thickened. Two important points have to be considered:

- The duodenum is very fragile and usually inflamed, especially in gastric outlet obstruction. Care should be taken to avoid crushing it with the linear cutter. If possible the cutter should be applied once, closed, and then fired. Several applications of the cutter without firing will only destroy the various layers and increase the risk of a duodenal stump leak.
- Sometimes the use of a 30-mm cutter is recommended for laparoscopic GI surgery. Here, it is advisable to use one firing of a 60-mm cutter because the duodenum is not an easy organ to handle with cutters, and it is difficult to cross staple lines on the duodenum.

Once the duodenum is transected, the stomach can be pulled upward and the lesser curvature is skeletonized. The posterior attachments of the stomach to the pancreas are divided, thus allowing full mobilization of the stomach.

Two anastomotic techniques exist for creation of the gastrojejunostomy: intra-abdominal gastrojejunostomy and laparoscopically-assisted gastrojejunostomy.

■ **Intra-abdominal Gastrojejunostomy and Billroth II Reconstruction.** There are two technical variants. After gastric transection with the linear cutters, the specimen may be removed through a 3 cm muscle splitting incision using one of the trocar sites (Fig. 6.8a). Alternatively the specimen may be left in place, the jejunal loop stapled on the posterior aspect of the stomach, and the specimen resected after the gastrojejunostomy has been performed (Fig. 6.8b). Whatever the choice, it is advisable to use several firings of a 30-mm cutter rather than a single firing of a 60-mm cutter which is bulky and more difficult to handle in this instance. Green staples are preferable on the thickened stomach.

When the gastrojejunostomy is complete, the two enterotomies are closed either with the specimen in place or the specimen resected and removed,. This is best done using intracorporeal suturing techniques with a running 3–0 Prolene suture (Fig. 6.9). This is preferable to the application of linear cutters that could narrow the anastomosis. It is also a good idea to leave the nasogastric tube in the jejunal loop to calibrate the loop and avoid any bites in the posterior wall while suturing the gastrotomies and enterotomies.

■ **Laparoscopic Gastrojejunostomy and Roux-en-Y Reconstruction.** Possibly, a better way to reconstruct is to create a 70 cm Roux-en-Y. It is created in the same fashion described in the technique of Roux-en-Y gastric bypass in the bariatric surgery chapter, and the gastrojejunal anastomosis is performed as described above.

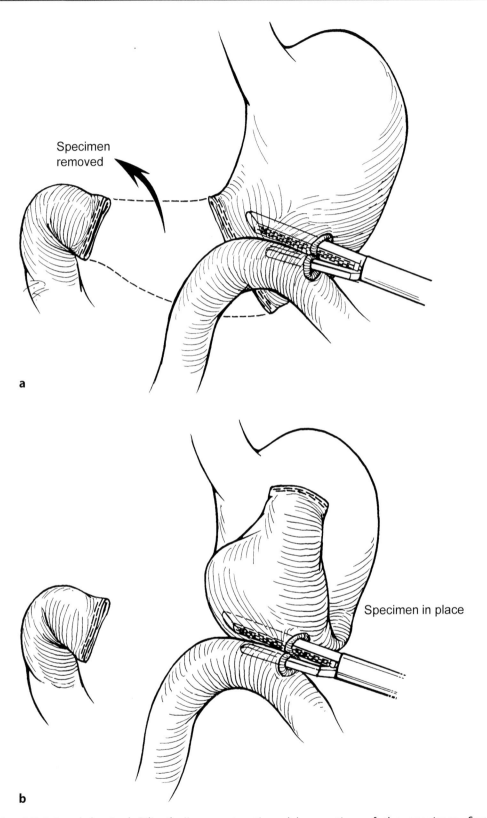

Fig. 6.8 Intra-abdominal Biliroth II reconstruction: (**a**) resection of the specimen first; (**b**) Biliroth II reconstruction first, specimen in place

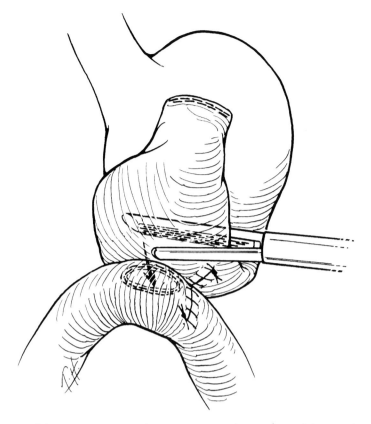

Fig. 6.9 Closure of the gastrotomy and enterotomy and resection of the specimen

■ **Laparoscopically-Assisted Gastrojejunostomy.** This is the author's preferred technique. It is more straightforward and requires no greater muscle incision than that for removal of the specimen. The rationale is to exteriorize the stomach and jejunum through a 3 cm muscle splitting incision in the left rectus muscle by enlarging the 10 mm trocar port used for the introduction of the instruments.

To inspect the bowel and pick up the jejunal loop, the surgeon moves to the right side of the patient, who is put in the Trendelenburg position. This will expose the small bowel, while the assistant retracts upward on the transverse colon. The jejunal loop that will be exteriorized is marked with endoclips for identification: this can be one small mark proximally and two marks distally (Fig. 6.10). The Bilroth II is then performed as in open surgery and the stomach is replaced in the abdomen (Fig. 6.11).

At the conclusion of the procedure there are two useful final steps. First, until the surgeon gains experience with this operation, the stomach should be checked for leaks by filling it with methylene blue and inflating. Second, placing the patient in a Trendelenburg position ensures that all fluids are collected above the mesocolon and aspirated, as some enteral fluid may remain and promote abscess creation in the postoperative period.

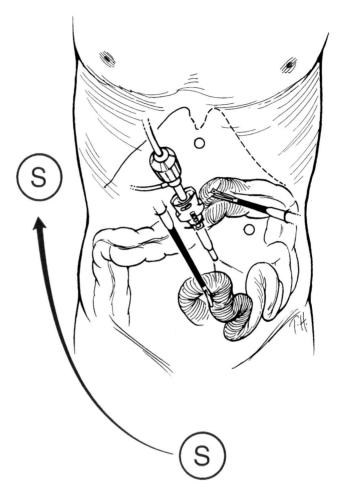

Fig. 6.10 Exposure of the jejunum in gastrectomy. The surgeon (*S*) moves to the right side of the patient and the scope is oriented down towards the pelvis

Perforated Duodenal Ulcer

If the patient's condition is stable, and peritonitis is diagnosed within 12 h of onset, it is possible to perform an operation laparoscopically (after 12 h, chemical peritonitis will give way to bacterial peritonitis presenting with severe sepsis, and laparoscopy may not be recommended in this situation). Care should be taken not to use a high insufflation pressure which could push intra-abdominal bacteria into the blood stream leading to bacteremia and septic shock. Pneumoperitoneum pressure should be maintained below 11 mmHg.

Locating the Perforation

Pneumoperitoneum is created in the traditional way. Four ports are then inserted using the triangulation concept, to form a diamond-shape. The surgeon stands between the legs of the patient, with the first assistant to the right and a second assistant to the left. The lead surgeon thus works comfortably with two hands, triangulated between the cameras (Fig. 6.12).

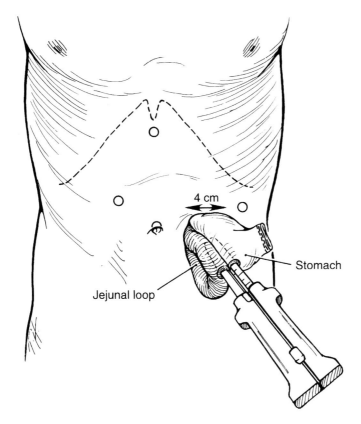

Fig. 6.11 Exteriorization of the stomach and jejunum for side-to-side stapled Biliroth II gastrojejunostomy

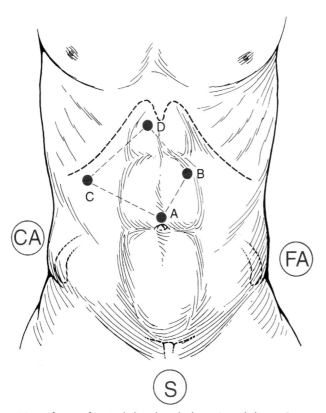

Fig. 6.12 Port positions for perforated duodenal ulcer. *A* umbilicus; *B* surgeon's right hand; *C* surgeon's left hand, *D* irrigation and suction and/or fan retractor for liver retraction. *S* surgeon; *FA* first assistant; *CA* camera assistant

The gallbladder, which usually adheres to the perforation, is retracted by the surgeon's left hand and moved upwards. The gallbladder is passed to the assistant using the subxyphoid port, which is placed to the right of the falciform ligament. The exposed area is checked and the perforation is usually clearly identified as a pinpoint hole on the anterior aspect of the duodenum, which has been covered by the fundus of the gallbladder. If the perforation is larger than the tip of the irrigation suction device (7–8 mm) and the crater is inflamed and friable, it is recommended to convert to an open procedure to safely close the perforation following a Kocher maneuver.

Abdominal Washout

The next step is careful and thorough irrigation and suction of all the intra-abdominal fluid. This should be done before the closure of the perforation to avoid any inadvertent disruption of the sutures during the washout. This is a tedious but essential task and needs *patience*. To irrigate and aspirate the whole abdomen requires about 10 L of saline mixed with local antibiotics.

Each quadrant is cleaned methodically, starting at the right upper quadrant, going to the left, moving down to the left lower quadrant, and then finally over to the right. Special attention should be given to the vesicorectal pouch. Fibrous membranes are removed as much as possible, since they may contain bacteria. The use of a 2 × 2 gauze introduced through one of the ports is helpful. However, if taking out fibrin attachments means injuring the intra-abdominal viscus, it should be done conservatively. This is a judgment call.

Management of the upper quadrants requires the surgeon to stand between the patient's legs. For the lower quadrants the surgeon should move to the right side of the patient, who should be tilted in Trendelenburg to give access to the pelvis. Special care should be taken to irrigate and aspirate between the loops of the small bowel. Once all this has been done, the patient is tilted back to the normal position for the surgeon to close the perforation.

Closure of the Perforation with an Omental Patch

The perforation is closed using an omental patch (Fig. 6.13).

An intracorporeal technique is preferred to avoid undue tension on the closure. It is advisable to insert the omental patch in the knot (*true Graham patch*), rather than use the tails of the knot to fix the patch as a result of which a small space remains between the knot itself and the omental patch, thereby diminishing the efficacy of the patch (Fig. 6.14a, b). The classic technique follows the same rules as with the original open Graham patch. The assistant holds the omental patch while the surgeon uses both hands to knot the ties. It is not necessary to place an abdominal drain if the procedure has been conducted appropriately.

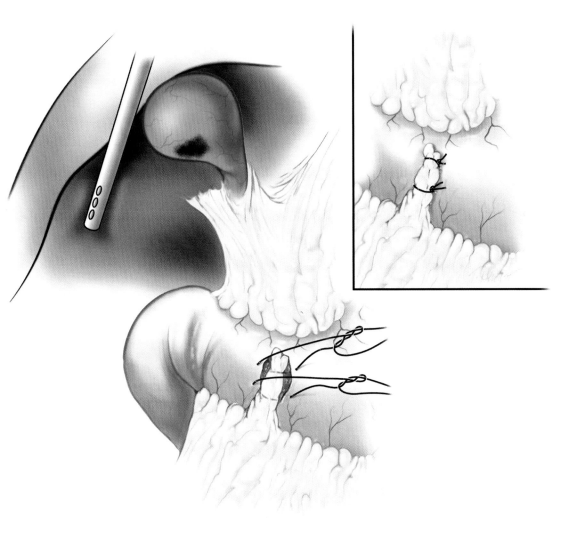

Fig. 6.13 Closure of the perforation

Postoperative Course

The patient ambulates the next day and liquids are started in moderation on the third day; if the vitals are normal and there is no sepsis, the patient is discharged on an anti-helicobacter regimen for 14 days starting that day. We do not routinely order a gastrographin swallow.

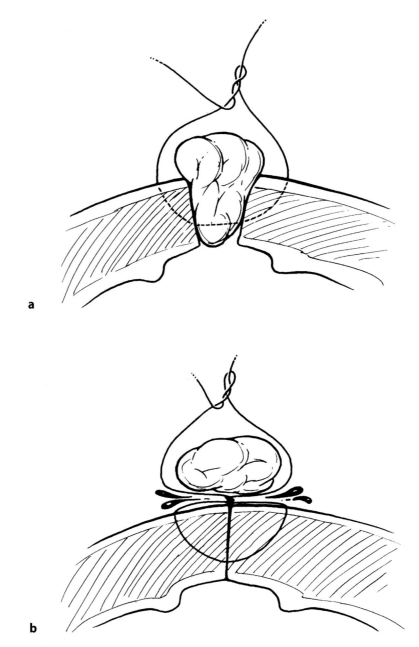

a

b

Fig. 6.14 Omental patches: (**a**) a patch plugging the hole between the threads of the stitch, and (**b**) a less efficacious arrangement with the patch between the tails of the tied knots

Anvari M, Park A (1994) Laparoscopic-assisted vagotomy and distal gastrectomy. Surg Endosc 8(11):1312–1315

Ballesta-Lopez C, Bastida-Vila X, Catarci M, Mato R, Ruggiero R (1996) Laparoscopic Billroth II distal subtotal gastrectomy with gastric stump suspension for gastric malignancies. Am J Surg 171(2):289–292

Champault GG (1994) Laparoscopic treatment of perforated peptic ulcer. Endosc Surg Allied Technol 2(2):117–118

Eypasch E, Stuttmann R, Jahn M, Troidl H, Doehn M (1995) Anesthesia for laparoscopic closure of perforated peptic ulcer–any harm or benefit? Endosc Surg Allied Technol 3(4):171–173

Fujita T (2009) Open or laparoscopic resection of a large gastric gastrointestinal stromal tumor. Arch Surg 144(2):193–194

Gagner M, Pomp A (1994) Laparoscopic pylorus-preserving pancreatoduodenectomy. Surg Endosc 8(5):408–410

Geis WP, Baxt R, Kim HC (1996) Benign gastric tumors. Minimally invasive approach. Surg Endosc 10(4):407–410

Goh PMY, Tekant Y, Kum CK et al (1992) Total intraabdominal laparoscopic Billroth II gastrectomy. Surg Endosc 6:160

Huguet KL, Rush RM Jr, Tessier DJ, Schlinkert RT, Hinder RA, Grinberg GG, Kendrick ML, Harold KL (2008) Laparoscopic gastric gastrointestinal stromal tumor resection: the mayo clinic experience. Arch Surg 143(6):587–590

Hwang SH, Park do J, Jee YS, Kim MC, Kim HH, Lee HJ, Yang HK, Lee KU (2009) Actual 3-year survival after laparoscopy-assisted gastrectomy for gastric cancer. Arch Surg 144(6):559–564

Jagot P, Sauvanet A, Berthoux L, Beighiti J (1996) Laparoscopic mobilization of the stomach for oesophageal replacement. Br J Surg 83(4):540–542

Jeong GA, Cho GS, Kim HH, Lee HJ, Ryu SW, Song KY (2009) Laparoscopy-assisted total gastrectomy for gastric cancer: a multicenter retrospective analysis. Surgery 146(3):469–474

Johanet H, Cossa JP, Hamdan M, Marmuse JP, LeGoff JY, Benhamou G (1994) Laparoscopic gastrectomy for obstructing duodenal ulcer. J Laparoendosc Surg 4(6):447–450

Johansson B, Hallerback B, Glise H, Johnsson B (1996) Laparoscopic suture closure of perforated peptic ulcer. A nonrandomized comparison with open surgery. Surg Endosc 10(6):656–658

Kaiser AM, Katkhouda N (2002) Laparoscopic management of perforated viscus. Semin Laparosc Surg 9:46–53

Katkhouda N (1994) Peptic ulcer surgery in 1994. Endosc Surg New Technol 2:7–9

Katkhouda N (1995) Laparoscopic treatment on gastroesophageal reflux disease; defining a gold standard. Surg Endosc 9:765–767

Katkhouda N, Mouiel J (1991) A new technique of surgical treatment of chronic duodenal ulcer without laparotomy by videocoelioscopy. Am J Surg 161:361–369

Katkhouda N, Iovine L, Mouiel J (1993) Right vagotomy and anterior fundic seromyotomy in the treatment of non complicated duodenal ulcer. J Coeliosurg 7:5–9 (in French)

Katkhouda N, Heimbucher J, Mouiel J (1994a) Laparoscopic posterior vagotomy and anterior seromyotomy. Endosc Surg New Technol 2:95–99

Katkhouda N, Heimbucher J, Mouiel J (1994b) Laparoscopic posterior truncal vagotomy and anterior seromyotomy. Semin Laparosc Surg 13:154–160

Katkhouda N, Waldrep D, Campos G, Offerman ST, Trussler A (1998) Laparoscopic highly selective vagotomy using the harmonic shears on improved technique. Surg Endosc 12:1051–1054

Katkhouda N, Mavor E, Mason R, Campos GMR, Soroushyari A, Berne TV (1999) Laparoscopic repair of perforated duodenal ulcers. Arch Surg 134:845–850

Katkhouda N, Friedlander M, Grant S, Mavor E, Achanta K, Essani R, Mouiel J (2000) Laparoscopic repair of intrathoracic volvulus. Surgery 128:784–790

Kim W, Song KY, Lee HJ, Han SU, Hyung WJ, Cho GS (2008) The impact of comorbidity on surgical outcomes in laparoscopy-assisted distal gastrectomy: a retrospective analysis of multicenter results. Ann Surg 248(5):793–799

Kitano S, Iso Y, Moriyama M, Sugimachi K (1994) Laparoscopy-assisted Billroth I gastrectomy. Surg Laparosc Endosc 4(2):146–148

Kojima K, Yamada H, Inokuchi M, Kawano T, Sugihara K (2008) A comparison of Roux-en-Y and Billroth-I reconstruction after laparoscopy-assisted distal gastrectomy. Ann Surg 247(6):962–967

Lau WY, Leung KL, Zhu XL, Lam YH, Chung SC, Li AK (1995) Laparoscopic repair of perforated peptic ulcer. Br J Surg 82(6):814–816

Lau WY, Leung KL, Kwong KH et al (1996) A randomized study comparing laparoscopic versus open repair of perforated peptic ulcer using suture or sutureless technique. Ann Surg 224(2):131–138

Liakakos T, Roukos DH (2009) Randomized evidence for laparoscopic gastrectomy short-term quality of life improvement and challenges for improving long-term outcomes. Ann Surg 250(2):349–350

Liorente J (1994) Laparoscopic gastric resection for gastric leiomyoma. Surg Endosc 8(8):887

Lord RV, Huprich JE, Katkhouda N (2000) Images of interest. Gastrointestinal: complications of fundoplication. J Gastroenterol Hepatol 15:1221

Mason RJ, Lipham J, Eckerling G, Schwartz A, Demeester TR (2005) Gastric electrical stimulation: an alternative surgical therapy for patients with gastroparesis. Arch Surg 140(9):841–846

Matsuda M, Nishiyama M, Hanai T, Saeki S, Watanabe T (1995) Laparoscopic omental patch repair for perforated peptic ulcer. Ann Surg 221(3):236–240

Memon MA (1995) Laparoscopic omental patch repair for perforated peptic ulcer. Ann Surg 222(6):761–762

Miserez M, Eypasch E, Spangenberger W, Lefering R, Troidl H (1996) Laparoscopic and conventional closure of perforated peptic ulcer. A comparison. Surg Endosc 10(8):831–836

Mouiel J, Katkhouda N (1991) Laparoscopic vagotomy in the treatment of chronic duodenal ulcer disease. Prob Gen Surg 83:358–365

Mouiel J, Katkhouda N (1993) Laparoscopic vagotomy for chronic duodenal ulcer. World J Surg 7:34–39

Mouiel J, Katkhouda N, Gugenheim J, Fabiani P, Goubaux B (1990) Treatment of duodenal ulcer by posterior truncal vagotomy and anterior fundic seromyotomy by video-coeliocopy. Preliminary results. Chirurgie 116:546–551 (in French)

Mouiel J, Katkhouda N, Gugenheim J, Fabiani P, DiMarzo L, Bertrandy M (1991) Elective laparoscopic surgery in duodenal ulcer. La Lettre Chir 8:100

Mouiel J, Katkhouda N, Gugenheim J, Fabiani P (1995) Posterior truncal vagotomy and seromyotomy by laparoscopy. J Coeliosurg 15:53–57 (in French)

Otani Y, Furukawa T, Yoshida M, Saikawa Y, Wada N, Ueda M, Kubota T, Mukai M, Kameyama K, Sugino Y, Kumai K, Kitajima M (2006) Operative indications for relatively small (2-5 cm) gastrointestinal stromal tumor of the stomach based on analysis of 60 operated cases. Surgery 139(4):484–492

So JB, Kum CK, Fernandes ML, Goh P (1996) Comparison between laparoscopic and conventional omental patch repair for perforated duodenal ulcer. Surg Endosc 10(11):1060–1063

Soper NJ, Brunt LM, Brewer JD, Meininger TA (1994) Laparoscopic Billroth II gastrectomy in the canine model. Surg Endosc 8(12):1395–1398

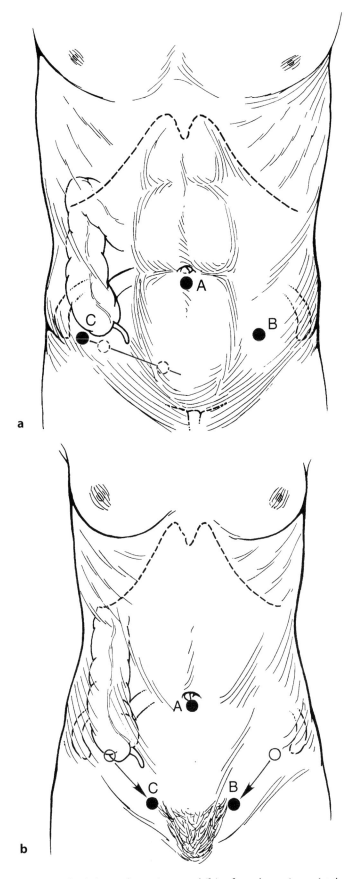

Fig. 7.2 Port positions for (**a**) a male patient and (**b**) a female patient. *A* telescope; *B* surgeon's right hand; *C* surgeon's left hand

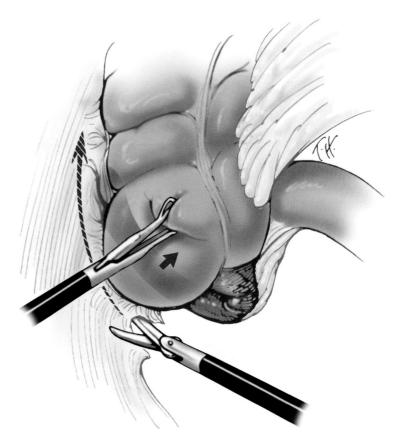

Fig. 7.3 Mobilization of the cecum in the event of a retrocecal appendix

Technique

There are two possible techniques that can be used to divide the appendix and mesoappendix: an endoloop technique or a stapling technique.

■ **Endoloop Technique.** The adhesions from the appendix to the surrounding organs and the mesentery are divided using the harmonic scalpel or bipolar forceps. The base of the appendix is identified next. Two endoloops are inserted and tied at the base. Another loop is then inserted next to the first two loops and the appendix is transected between the two proximal loops and the distal loop. Finally, the mucosa is cauterized (Fig. 7.4).

■ **Stapling Technique.** A window is created at the base of the mesoappendix and a 30-mm white vascular stapler inserted (Fig. 7.5). The mesoappendix is transected, followed by the base of the appendix, using a 30-mm blue stapler. The appendix is cut as close as possible to the cecum leaving a very short stump. The mesentery and base of the appendix are checked for any evidence of bleeding. If bleeding is present from staple line, it should be controlled by placing a clip. The appendix is placed in a bag and removed from the abdomen. Alternatively, if the appendix is thin, it can be pulled into the port and withdrawn with it, so the wound is not contaminated.

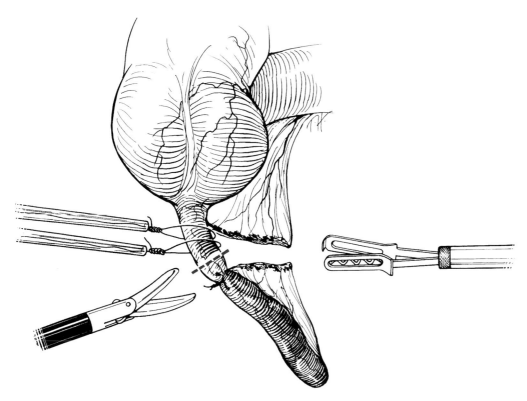

Fig. 7.4 Endoloop technique in appendectomy

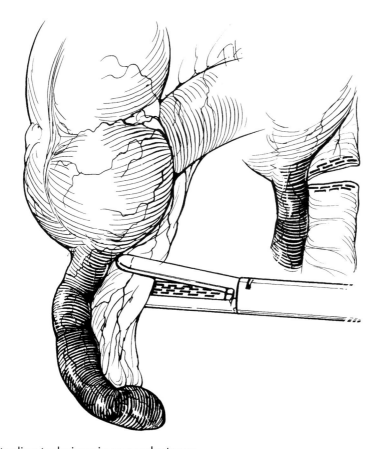

Fig. 7.5 Stapling technique in appendectomy

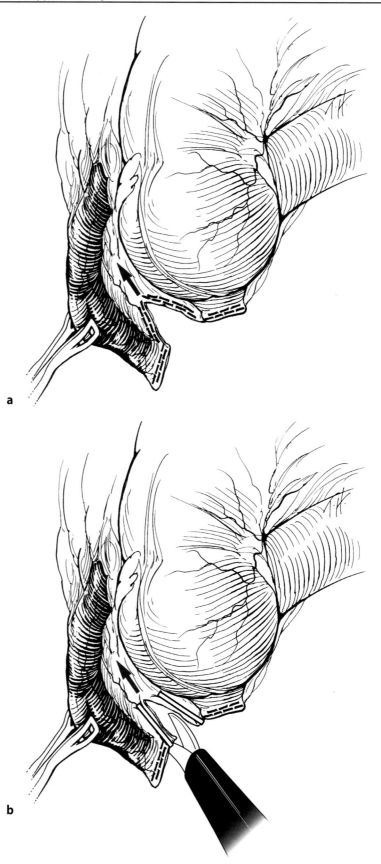

Fig. 7.6 (**a**) Retrograde appendectomy when the tip of the appendix is not visible (base→ tip), using firings of the stapler. (**b**) Retrograde appendectomy using clips and scissors ("clip-cut" technique)

If the tip of the appendix is not clearly visible, a retrograde appendectomy can be performed using the stapler (Fig. 7.6a). The visible base of the appendix is transected after creation of an appropriate window, followed by the mesoappendix, and finally the whole appendix is dissected out from the base to the tip. This is done as in open surgery and does not require specific skills. It is also possible to utilize the "clip-cut" technique (Fig. 7.6b). This is especially useful in a case of retrocecal appendicitis. The base of the appendix is stapled; clips are placed on the mesentery, and more clips are then placed until the tip of the appendix is completely mobilized. With the appendix removed, care is taken to perform thorough suctioning of the area without much irrigation, so that a drain is not necessary.

Gangrenous or Perforated Appendicitis

When the surgeon encounters an appendiceal phlegmon, it can be difficult to identify the appendix. In these circumstances, it may be necessary to mobilize the cecum first. This mobilization should be as conservative as possible so as not to open retroperitoneal spaces that might be contaminated (Fig. 7.3).

The cecum can then be flipped over and the appendix visualized. If this is still not possible, the only way forward is to convert to an open operation. The projection of the cecum is marked on the abdominal wall using transillumination of the laparoscope, and a corresponding incision is then made.

Alternatively, in difficult circumstances it is possible to remove the port from the right lower quadrant and insert a finger in the opening to perform an atraumatic mobilization of the cecum under laparoscopic guidance (Fig. 7.7a, b). This *"fingeroscopy"* technique allows blunt dissection of a phlegmon when it is difficult to define healthy bowel from necrotic tissue. It will speed the procedure and restore tactile feeling. It should be considered as the last step in situations where conversion seems inevitable. The combined use of the irrigation and suction device and the finger is particularly useful to break the loculations and aspirate the pus.

The greater hazard of laparoscopic appendectomy is the possibility of residual intraabdominal infection leading to pelvis abscess. This is especially true in the case of perforated or suppurative appendicitis. Figure 7.8 depicts the maneuver for irrigation of the pelvis in open surgery. The problem is that some of the infected irrigation fluid is left behind in the pelvis, further contributing to the risk of pelvic abscess. To aspirate the cul de sac under direct vision, a specific maneuver is required. The patient is placed in Trendelenberg position and the surgeon who was looking to the right side now looks at the pelvis (Fig. 7.9). Using both trocars, the sigmoid colon is retracted with the left hand, thus exposing the cul de sac (Fig. 7.10); irrigation is performed and all the fluid is sucked under direct vision (Fig. 7.11). This maneuver will dramatically reduce the risk of intra abdominal abscess especially in the pelvis. The supra-hepatic area is also checked for the presence of purulent fluid that needs to be suctioned.

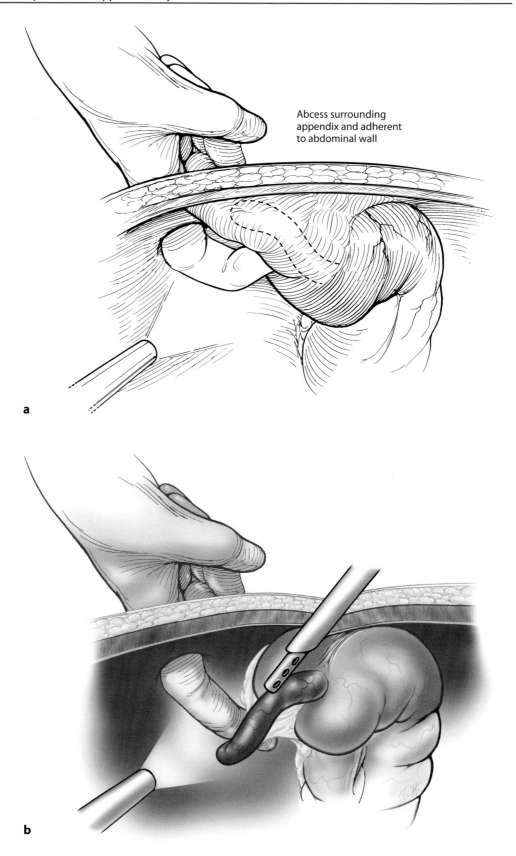

Abcess surrounding
appendix and adherent
to abdominal wall

a

b

Fig. 7.7 (**a**) "Fingeroscopy": finger inserted in the trocar incision and breaking up a loculated abscess. (**b**) "Fingeroscopy": demonstrating the combined use of the finger and the suction irrigation device

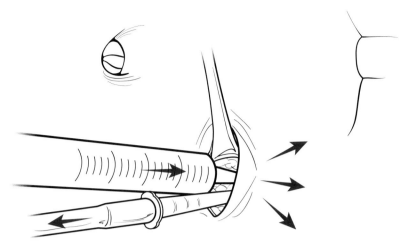

Fig. 7.8 Classic irrigation technique in open appendectomy for perforated appendicitis, possibly leaving behind some infected fluid in the pelvis, leading to pelvic abscess

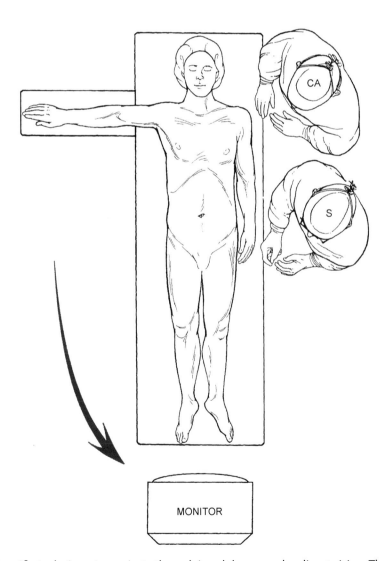

Fig. 7.9 Specific technique to aspirate the pelvic cul de sac under direct vision. The monitor is moved to the feet, where the surgeon then looks

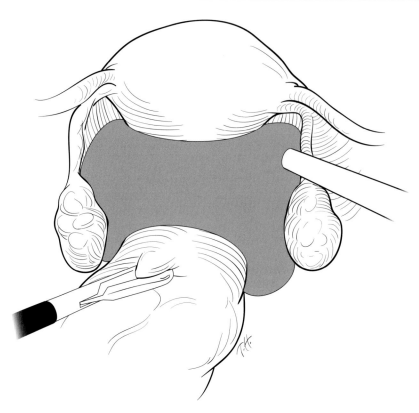

Fig. 7.10 To aspirate the cul de sac under direct vision, the sigmoid colon is retracted with the left hand, and the irrigation device is placed in the pelvis

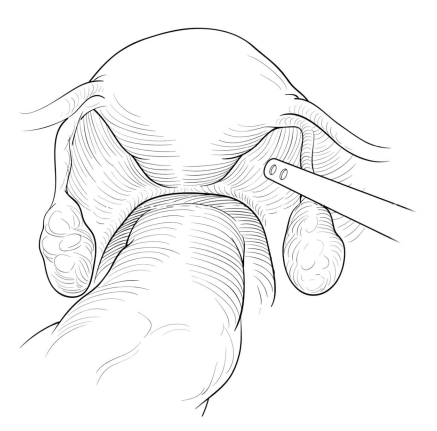

Fig. 7.11 Aspiration of infected fluid under direct vision

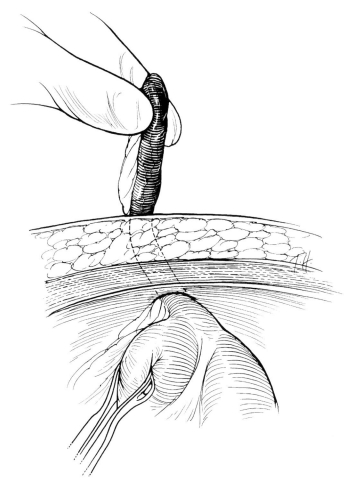

Fig. 7.12 Laparoscopically-assisted appendectomy (useful in pediatric appendectomy)

In some cases, especially in children, where the appendix is extremely long and the working space small, the laparoscopic "assisted" technique is an easy way of performing an appendectomy.

The mesoappendix is first controlled with a harmonic scalpel. Next, the port is removed with the appendix inside. The entire appendix is exteriorized and ligated outside the abdomen before the cecum is pushed back inside the abdomen (Fig. 7.12).

Care is needed to avoid infecting or contaminating the abdomen. For this reason, maneuvers should be minimized while pulling the appendix out of the incision.

Laparoscopic Assisted Appendectomy

Selected Further Reading

Des Groseilliers S, Fortin M, Lokanathan R, Khoury N, Mutch D (1995) Laparoscopic appendectomy versus open appendectomy: retrospective assessment of 200 patients. Can J Surg 38(2):178–182

El-Ghoneimi A, Valla JS, Limonne B et al (1994) Laparoscopic appendectomy in children: report of 1,379 cases. J Pediatr Surg 29(6):786–789

Faiz O, Clark J, Brown T, Bottle A, Antoniou A, Farrands P, Darzi A, Aylin P (2008) Traditional and laparoscopic appendectomy in adults: outcomes in English NHS hospitals between 1996 and 2006. Ann Surg 248(5):800–806

Fujita T (2009) Is laparoscopic appendectomy associated with better outcomes? Ann Surg 249(5):867

Fujita T, Yanaga K (2007) Appendectomy: negative appendectomy no longer ignored. Arch Surg 142(11):1023–1025

Frazee RC, Bohannon WT (1996) Laparoscopic appendectomy for complicated appendicitis. Arch Surg 131(5):509–511

Frazee RC, Roberts JW, Symmonds RE et al (1994) A prospective randomized trial comparing open versus laparoscopic appendectomy. Ann Surg 219(6):725–728

Gotz F, Pier A, Bacher C (1990) Modified laparoscopic appendicectomy in surgery. A report on 388 operations. Surg Endosc 4:6–9

Hale DA, Molloy M, Pearl RH, Schutt DC, Jaques DP (1997) Appendectomy: a contemporary appraisal. Ann Surg 225(3):252–261

Hansen JB, Smithers BM, Schache D, Wall DR, Miller BJ, Menzies BL (1996) Laparoscopic versus open appendectomy: prospective randomized trial. World J Surg 20(1):17–20

Heinzelmann M, Simmen HP, Cummins AS, Largiader F (1995) Is laparoscopic appendectomy the new "gold standard"? Arch Surg 130(7):782–785

Ikard RW, Federspiel CF (1995) Laparoscopic versus open appendectomy. N Engl J Med 333(13):881–882

Katkhouda N, Mason RJ, Towfigh S, Gevorgyan A, Essani R (2005) Laparoscopic versus open appendectomy: a prospective randomized double-blind study. Ann Surg 242(3):439–448

Katkhouda N, Friedlander M, Grant S, Achanta K, Essani MR, Paik P, Campos G, Mason R, Mavor E (2000) Intra-abdominal abscess rate following laparoscopic appendectomy. Am J Surg 180:456–459

Katkhouda N, Mavor E, Campos G, Mason R, Waldrep D (1999) Finger assisted laparoscopy (fingeroscopy) for treatment of complicated appendicitis. J Am Coll Surg 189:130–133

Kluiber RM, Hartsman B (1996) Laparoscopic appendectomy. A comparison with open appendectomy. Dis Colon Rectum 39(9):1008–1011

Kollias J, Harries RH, Otto G, Hamilton DW, Cox JS, Gallery RM (1994) Laparoscopic versus open appendectomy for suspected appendicitis: a prospective study. Aust N Z J Surg 64(12):830–835

Leung TT, Dixon E, Gill M, Mador BD, Moulton KM, Kaplan GG, MacLean AR (2009) Bowel obstruction following appendectomy: what is the true incidence? Ann Surg 250(1):51–53

Lujan-Mompean JA, Robles-Campos R, Parrilla-Paricio P, Soria-Aledo V, Garcia-Ayllon J (1994) Laparoscopic versus open appendectomy: a prospective assessment. Br J Surg 81(1):133–135

Lukish J, Powell D, Morrow S, Cruess D, Guzzetta P (2007) Laparoscopic appendectomy in children: use of the endoloop vs the endostapler. Arch Surg 142(1):58–61

McCahill LE, Pellegrini CA, Wiggins T, Helton WS (1996) A clinical outcome and cost analysis of laparoscopic versus open appendectomy. Am J Surg 171(5):533–537

Martin LC, Puente I, Sosa JL et al (1995) Open versus laparoscopic appendectomy. A prospective randomized comparison. Ann Surg 222(3):256–261

Neugebauer E, Troidi H, Kum CK, Eypasch E, Miserez M, Paul A (1995) The E.A.E.S. Consensus Development Conferences on laparoscopic cholecystectomy, appendectomy, and hernia repair. Consensus statements September 1994. The Educational Committee of the European Association for Endoscopic Surgery. Surg Endosc 9(5):550–563

Ortega AE, Hunter JG, Peters JH, Swanstrom LL, Schirmer B (1995) A prospective, randomized comparison of laparoscopic appendectomy with open appendectomy. Laparoscopic Appendectomy Study Group. Am J Surg 169(2):208–212

Richards KF, Fisher KS, Flores JH, Christensen BJ (1996) Laparoscopic appendectomy: com parison with open appendectomy in 720 patients. Surg Laparosc Endosc 6(3):205–209

Sleem R, Fisher S, Gestring M, Cheng J, Sangosanya A, Stassen N, Bankey P (2009) Perforated appendicitis: is early laparoscopic appendectomy appropriate? Surgery 146(4):731–737

Somerville PU, Lavelle MA (1996) Residual appendicitis following incomplete laparoscopic appendectomy. Br J Surg 83(6):869

Tang E, Ortega AE, Anthone GJ, Beart RW Jr (1996) Intraabdominal abscesses following laparoscopic and open appendectomies. Surg Endosc 10(3):327–328

Tate JJ (1996) Laparoscopic appendectomy. Br J Surg 83(9):1169–1170

Towfigh S, Formosa C, Katkhouda N, Kelso R, Sohn H, Berne T (2008) Obesity should not influence management of appendicitis. Surg Endosc 22:2601–2605

Towfigh S, Chen F, Mason R, Katkhouda N, Chan L, Berne T (2006) Laparoscopic appendectomy significantly reduces length of stay for perforated appendicitis. Surg Endosc 20:495–499

Wagner M, Aronsky D, Tschudi J, Metzger A, Klaiber C (1996) Laparoscopic stapler appendectomy. A prospective study of 267 consecutive cases. Surg Endosc 10(9):895–899

Varela JE, Hinojosa MW, Nguyen NT (2008) Laparoscopy should be the approach of choice for acute appendicitis in the morbidly obese. Am J Surg 196(2):218–222

Zaninotto G, Rossi M, Anselmino M et al (1995) Laparoscopic versus conventional surgery for suspected appendicitis in women. Surg Endosc 9(3):337–340

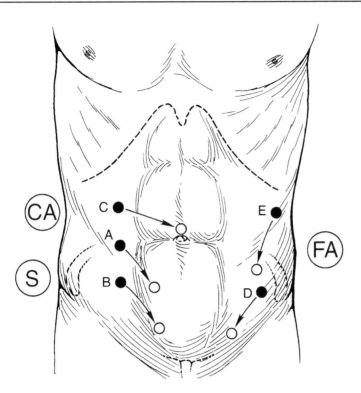

Fig. 8.4 Port positions for left colectomy (note that all trocars are moved down for low anterior resection, as in Fig. 8.5). *A* surgeon's left hand; *B* surgeon's right hand, also used for the introduction of the stapler; *C* camera; *D, E* graspers of the assistant. *S* surgeon; *FA* first assistant; *CA* camera assistant

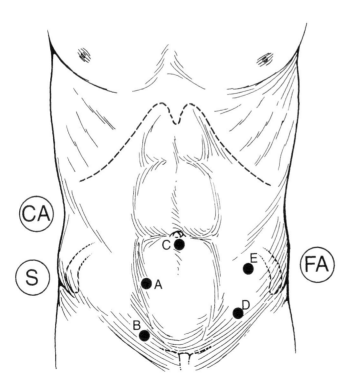

Fig. 8.5 Port positions for low anterior resection (Fig. 8.4). *A* surgeon's left hand; *B* surgeon's right hand, also used for the introduction of the stapler; *C* camera; *D, E* graspers of the assistant. *S* surgeon; *FA* first assistant; *CA* camera assistant

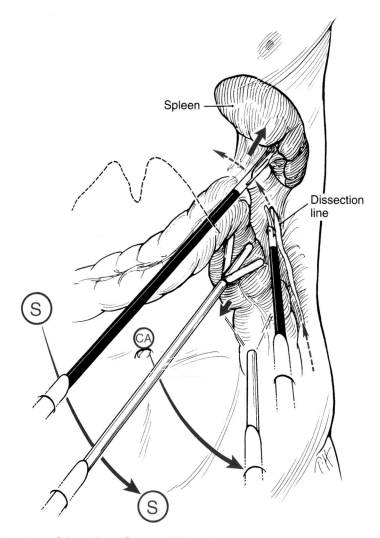

Fig. 8.6 Dissection of the splenic flexure of the colon. *S* surgeon; *CA* camera assistant

resected tissue doughnuts to ensure that they are complete. An incomplete doughnut should prompt a laparoscopic suture repair of the anastomosis. If the area of the rupture is not recognized, the entire anastomosis should be revised and interrupted sutures placed around the circumference. Should this not be possible, the procedure is converted to an open operation.

In the medial to lateral approach, the sigmoid colon is grasped with the left hand and retracted until the superior hemorrhoidal arteries are under tension. A window is made around the vessels, and at this point the left ureter SHOULD be visualized before placement of the stapler. After the vessels are transected, the rest of the procedure is performed as described.

If a hand port is used, again it can be placed through a midline of a Pfannenstiel incision.

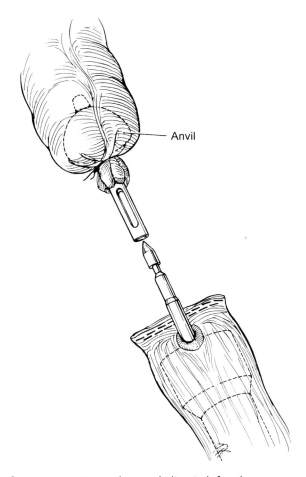

Fig. 8.7 Rectal perforation anterior to the staple line in left colectomy

The above comments relating to left colectomy also apply to the Hartmann procedure, except that there is no anastomosis and the mobilized colon is exteriorized through one of the port openings. A colostomy can then be performed at the site of the trocar orifice.

Hartmann Procedure

This operation is not difficult, provided there are not too many adhesions. The first step is to take down the colostomy. The colon is trimmed outside, and the anvil of the EEA stapler is introduced and secured with a purse string suture. Then the colostomy site is used for a Hasson port, and insufflation begins. Dense adhesions can block the view, and must be carefully dissected; this is especially true in the midline, as the adhesions obscure the view for the insertion of additional ports. The port sites must therefore be suitably chosen to permit lysis of adhesions (Fig. 8.8). Once the rectal stump has been pierced with the shaft of the circular stapler, an anastomosis is performed.

One possible problem in this operation is inadvertent stapling of the bladder, especially in male patients. It is therefore essential to check the bladder and to make sure that it is not involved in the suture line, as this will increase the risk of creating a colovesical fistula. Two maneuvers reduce the risk of bladder injury. Firstly, the bladder is inflated with saline through a Foley catheter to visualize the limits of the bladder; secondly, a metallic dilator is introduced into the rectum to help identify the rectal stump.

Reversing the Hartmann Procedure

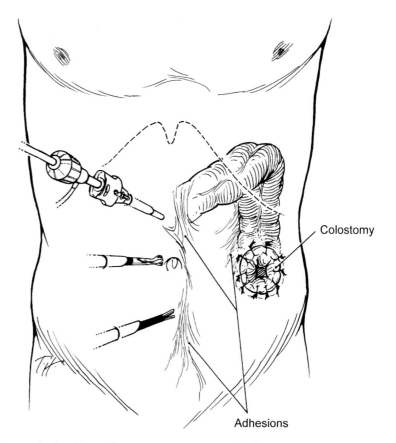

Fig. 8.8 Removal of midline adhesions prior to reversal of Hartmnann's procedure

Agachan F, Joo JS, Weiss EG, Wexner SD (1996) Intraoperative laparoscopic complications. Are we getting better? Dis Col Rec 39(10 suppl):S14–S19

Bardram L, Funch-Jensen P, Jensen P, Crawford ME, Kehlet H (1995) Recovery after laparoscopic colonic surgery with epidural analgesia, and early oral nutrition and mobilisation. Lancet 345(8952):763–764

Bilimoria KY, Bentrem DJ, Nelson H, Stryker SJ, Stewart AK, Soper NJ, Russell TR, Ko CY (2008) Use and outcomes of laparoscopic-assisted colectomy for cancer in the United States. Arch Surg 143(9):832–839; discussion 839–840

Bruce CJ, Coller JA, Murray JJ, Schoetz DJ Jr, Roberts PL, Rusin LC (1996) Laparoscopic resection for diverticular disease. Dis Colon Rectum 39(10 suppl):S1–S6

Clinical Outcomes of Surgical Therapy Study Group (2004) A comparison of laparoscopically assisted and open colectomy for colon cancer. N Engl J Med 350(20):2050–2059

Dalibon N, Moutafis M, Fischler M (2004) Laparoscopically assisted versus open colectomy for colon cancer. N Engl J Med 351(9):933–934

Fowler DL, White SA (1991) Laparoscopy-assisted sigmoid resection. Surg Laparosc Endosc 1:183–188

Franklin ME Jr, Rosenthal D, Abrego-Medina D et al (1996) Prospective comparison of open vs. laparoscopic colon surgery for carcinoma. Five-year results. Dis Colon Rectum 39(10 suppl):S35–S46

Gray MR, Curtis JM, Elkington JS (1994) Colovesical fistula after laparoscopic inguinal hernia repair. Br J Surg 81(8):1213–1214

Guillou PJ (1994) Laparoscopic surgery for diseases of the colon and rectum – quo vadis? Surg Endosc 8(6):669–671

Huscher C, Silecchia O, Croce E et al (1996) Laparoscopic colorectal resection. A multicenter Italian study. Surg Endosc 10(9):875–879

Lacy AM, Garcia-Valdecasas JC, Pique JM et al (1995) Short-term outcome analysis of a randomized study comparing laparoscopic vs open colectomy for colon cancer. Surg Endosc 9(10):1101–1105

Liberman MA, Phillips EH, Carroll BJ, Fallas M, Rosenthal R (1996) Laparoscopic colectomy vs traditional colectomy for diverticulitis. Outcome and costs. Surg Endosc 10(1):15–18

Lumley JW, Fielding GA, Rhodes M, Nathanson LK, Siu S, Stitz RW (1996) Laparoscopic assisted colorectal surgery. Lessons learned from 240 consecutive patients. Dis Colon Rectum 39(2):155–159

Mouiel J, Katkhouda N, Gugenheim J, Bloch J, Le Goff D, Benizri E, Darois J (1989) Near total colectomy followed by caeco-rectal anastomosis using stapling technique. Lyon Chir 85:192–194

Koopmann MC, Harms BA, Heise CP (2007) Money well spent: a comparison of hospital operating margin for laparoscopic and open colectomies. Surgery 142(4):546–553

Laurent C, Leblanc F, Wütrich P, Scheffler M, Rullier E (2009) Laparoscopic versus open surgery for rectal cancer: long-term oncologic results. Ann Surg 250(1):54–61

Pappas TN, Jacobs DO (2004) Laparoscopic resection for colon cancer–the end of the beginning? N Engl J Med 350(20):2091–2092

Ota DM (1995) Laparoscopic colon resection for cancer. Surg Endosc 9(12):1318–1322

Paik PS, Beart RW Jr (1997) Laparoscopic colectomy. Surg Clin N Am 77(1):1–13

Philipps EH, Franklin ME, Carroll BJ et al (1992) Laparoscopic colectomy. Ann Surg 216:703–707

Philipson BM, Bokey EL, Moore JW, Chapuis PH, Bagge E (1997) Cost of open versus laparoscopically assisted right hemicolectomy for cancer. World J Surg 21(2):214–217

Ramos JM, Gupta S, Anthone GJ, Ortega AE, Simons AJ, Beart RW Jr (1994) Laparoscopy and colon cancer. Is the port site at risk? A preliminary report. Arch Surg 129(9):897–899

Reissman P, Cohen S, Weiss EG, Wexner SD (1996) Laparoscopic colorectal surgery: ascending the learning curve. World J Surg 20(3):277–281

Sands LR, Wexner SD (1996) The role of laparoscopic colectomy and laparotomy with resection in the management of complex polyps of the colon. Surg Oncol Clin N Am 5(3):713–721

Stage JO, Schuize S, Moller P et al (1997) Prospective randomized study of laparoscopic versus open colonic resection for adenocarcinoma. Br J Surg 84(3):391–396

Teeuwen PH, Chouten MG, Bremers AJ, Bleichrodt RP (2009) Laparoscopic sigmoid resection for diverticulitis decreases major morbidity rates: a randomized controlled trial. Ann Surg 250(3):500–501

Velmahos G, Vassiliu P, Chan L, Murray J, Salim A, Demetriatdes D, Katkhouda N, Berne TV (2002) Wound management after colon injury: a prospective randomized trial. Am Surg 68:795–801

Veenhof AA, van der Peet DL, Cuesta MA (2009) Laparoscopic resection for diverticular disease: follow-up of 500 consecutive patients. Ann Surg 250(1):174–175

Wexner SD, Reissman P, Pfeifer J, Bernstein M, Geron N (1996) Laparoscopic colorectal surgery: analysis of 140 cases. Surg Endosc 10(2):133–136

Zucker KA, Pitcher DE, Martin DT, Ford RS (1994) Laparoscopic-assisted colon resection. Surg Endosc 8:12–17

Small Bowel Obstruction

9

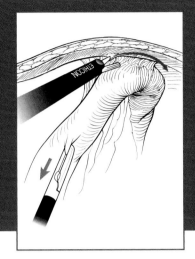

A patient presenting with small bowel obstruction in the presence of an abdominal scar, suggesting that an adhesive band may be present, is an ideal case for a laparoscopic approach.

The first step is localization of the site of the initial obstruction. This is accomplished by a thorough physical examination and imaging to identify the area of maximal bowel distention using a plain abdominal X-ray and a CT scan to find a transition point. The laparoscope is inserted on the side opposite to the site of maximal intestinal distension.

It is possible in these cases to perform an open Hasson technique and insert a blunt trocar providing direct viewing of the intra-abdominal contents. One can however use an alternative technique for inserting the first trocar. Making a small skin incision and opening the layers of the fascia under direct vision provides access to the abdomen. A purse string is placed on the fascia using 2–0 suture, and a 10-mm port together with a video laparoscope is inserted while the surgeon's left hand retracts the abdomen before insufflation. This allows the surgeon to visualize the intra-abdominal contents prior to insufflation, and ensures that the port and laparoscope are properly placed in the abdomen. The purse string is secured and insufflation is then begun, which generally puts the adhesive band under tension (Fig. 9.1).

Adequate working space is of paramount importance in the laparoscopic management of SBO. If the intra-abdominal pressure has reached a peak (15 mmHg) with the volume insufflated equal or less than 2 L, and provided the patient is well paralyzed, there is probably *not enough working space* due to the ileus. In this case, the operation should be converted to an open procedure.

N. Katkhouda, *Advanced Laparoscopic Surgery*,
DOI: 10.1007/978-3-540-74843-4_9, © Springer-Verlag Berlin Heidelberg 2011

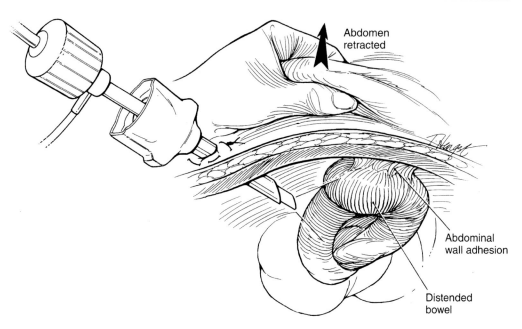

Abdomen
retracted

Abdominal
wall adhesion

Distended
bowel

Fig. 9.1 Laparoscopic enterolysis: alternative technique to the open Hasson approach, for the insertion of the first trocar

The table is then tilted in order to retract the small bowel and increase the working space. It is possible to position the patient in Trendelenburg or reverse Trendelenburg and with either side up in order to create the appropriate space.

Once pneumoperitoneum is created, any adhesive band can be directly visualized. Mobilization with the laparoscope itself by breaking some of the loose bands can make room for the insertion of the second port, which is usually the port for the surgeon's right hand when the surgeon is standing opposite the area of maximum abdominal distension.

Insertion of a second port permits introduction of scissors, which is the best instrument for laparoscopic enterolysis. When one is performing enterolysis, it is safer not to use electrocautery, and although the harmonic shear can facilitate dissection, a sharp dissection is the best. In the case of bowel stuck to the abdominal wall, it is possible to remove a piece of fascia with the small bowel (Fig. 9.2). This is certainly safer than trying to free the small bowel from the abdominal wall and exposing it to serosal tears or unrecognized injuries. If severe, dense adhesions are encountered, it is impossible to complete a dissection without violating the bowel, and it is best to convert to an open procedure.

Once the first two ports are inserted, it is possible to sharply dissect the adhesive band from the abdominal wall. It is best to stay close to the abdominal wall and at a respectable distance from the intra-abdominal contents to avoid injury. It is also recommended to limit the use of cautery; the harmonic shears are probably safer in this setting once enough working space is available.

The third and final port is inserted in a triangulated manner to the video laparoscope (Fig. 9.3). This is used to insert a grasper, allowing the left hand to put the adhesive band under tension while the right hand removes the attachment. This will allow mobilization of the small bowel. Harmonic scissors can be used for this part.

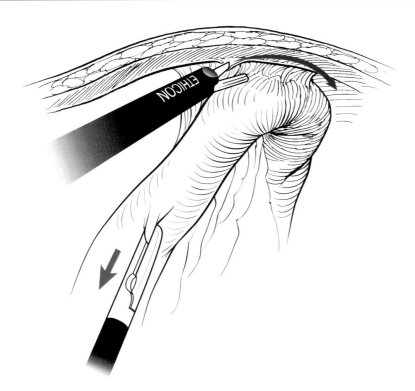

Fig. 9.2 Figure depicting the use of the harmonic shears for laparoscopic enterolysis and "shaving" the fascia, allowing it to stay on the small bowel to avoid a serosal or unrecognized injury to the small bowel

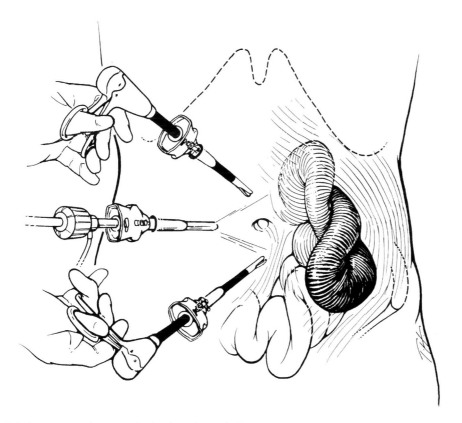

Fig. 9.3 Laparoscopic enterolysis: the triangulation concept

The best way to locate the adhesive band responsible for the obstruction is to follow the path of the small bowel and identify the junction between the dilated and nondilated portions of the bowel. This will lead immediately to the area of the stricture or obstruction. If the site of obstruction is not easily identified, locate the terminal ileum and run the bowel in a retrograde fashion to find the transition point. Occasionally if bowel is run anterograde, there is a chance that the band causing the obstruction is taken down, thereby decompressing the bowel without definitive localization of the band. When handling the bowel, great care is taken to avoid grasping the distended and paper-thin bowel wall with traumatic graspers. One should use the most atraumatic grasper possible (large fenestrated grapser).

Once the adhesive band has been removed, the small bowel should be inspected carefully to assess vascularity, motility, and the state of the serosa. If there is any doubt about the viability of the small bowel, an open inspection is mandatory. A small incision can be made, or one of the port incisions can be enlarged and the small bowel is examined outside the abdomen. If a resection is indicated, it can be performed extracorporeally, after which the bowel is carefully returned to the abdomen and the small incision closed.

Franklin ME Jr, Dorman JP, Pharand D (1994) Laparoscopic surgery in acute small bowel obstruction. Surg Laparosc Endosc 4(4):289–296

Gandhi AD, Patel RA, Brolin RE (2009) Elective laparoscopy for herald symptoms of mesenteric/internal hernia after laparoscopic Roux-en-Y gastric bypass. Surg Obes Relat Dis 5(2):144–149

Greig JD, Miles WF, Nixon SI (1995) Laparoscopic technique for small bowel biopsy. Br J Surg 82(3):363

Husain S, Ahmed AR, Johnson J, Boss T, O'Malley W (2007) Small-bowel obstruction after laparoscopic Roux-en-Y gastric bypass: etiology, diagnosis, and management. Arch Surg 142(10):988–993

Lange V, Meyer G, Schardey HM et al (1995) Different techniques of laparoscopic end-to-end small-bowel anastomoses. Surg Endosc 9(1):82–87

Lee IK, Kim do H, Gorden DL, Lee YS, Jung SE, Oh ST, Kim JG, Jeon HM, Kim EK, Chang SK (2009) Selective laparoscopic management of adhesive small bowel obstruction using CT guidance. Am Surg 75(3):227–231

Nagle A, Ujiki M, Denham W, Murayama K (2004) Laparoscopic adhesiolysis for small bowel obstruction. Am J Surg 187(4):464–470

Posta C (1996) Surgical decisions in the laparoscopic management of small bowel obstruction: report on two cases. J Laparoendosc Surg 6(2):117–120

Slutzki S, Halpern Z, Negri M, Kais H, Halevy A (1996) The laparoscopic second look for ischemic bowel disease. Surg Endosc 10(7):729–731

Waninger I, Salm R, Imdahl A et al (1996) Comparison of laparoscopic handsewn suture techniques for experimental small-bowel anastomoses. Surg Laparosc Endosc 6(4):282–289

Yau KK, Siu WT, Law BK, Cheung HY, Ha JP, Li MK (2005) Laparoscopic approach compared with conventional open approach for bezoar-induced small-bowel obstruction. Arch Surg 140(10):972–975

Zerey M, Sechrist CW, Kercher KW, Sing RF, Matthews BD, Heniford BT (2007) The laparoscopic management of small-bowel obstruction. Am J Surg 194(6):882–887

Selected Further Reading

Inguinal Hernia Repair 10

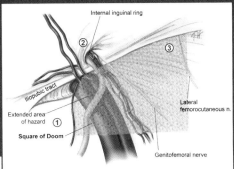

The understanding and recognition of the anatomy of the preperitoneal space is essential to the performance of a safe and effective laparoscopic hernia repair (Fig. 10.1). The five important landmarks are as follows:

General Considerations and Surgical Anatomy

1. Pubic tubercle and Cooper's ligament.
2. External iliac vein.
3. Medial umbilical ligament and the inferior epigastric vessels as they come off the external iliac vessels.
4. Vas deferens.
5. Cord vessels.

Along with the iliopubic tract, these landmarks define the three spaces associated with groin hernias (Fig. 10.2):

1. Indirect inguinal hernia: lateral to the inferior epigastric vessels.
2. Direct inguinal hernia: medial to the inferior epigastric vessels and lateral to the border of the rectus abdominus muscle within the triangle of Hesselbach.
3. Femoral hernia: under the iliopubic tract, medial to the iliac vein, and lateral to Cooper's ligament.

All three spaces should be covered by an appropriate size mesh. They are no different from the hernia spaces seen in the traditional open anterior approach (Fig. 10.3).

There are several dangerous areas of dissection with the laparoscopic repair. The "triangle of doom" is located between the vas deferens medially and the gonadal vessels

N. Katkhouda, *Advanced Laparoscopic Surgery*,
DOI: 10.1007/978-3-540-74843-4_10, © Springer-Verlag Berlin Heidelberg 2011

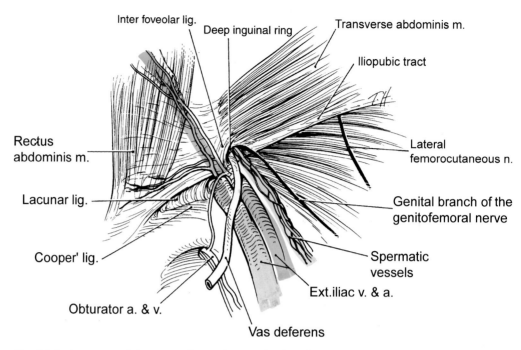

Fig. 10.1 Anatomy of the preperitoneal space (*right side*)

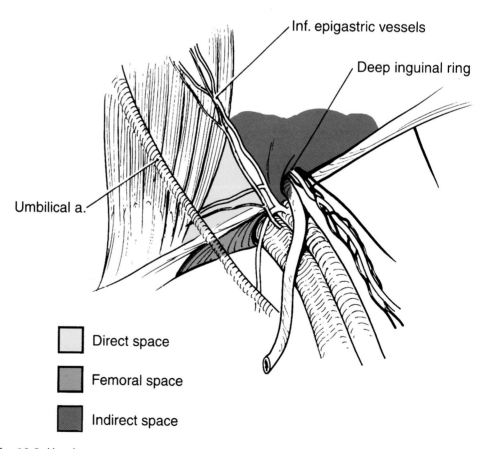

Fig. 10.2 Hernia spaces

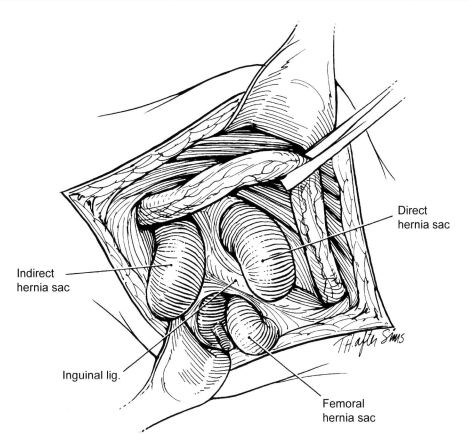

Fig. 10.3 Hernia spaces as seen from the anterior approach

laterally. The external iliac vein and artery are found in this triangle. There is another dangerous space at the superior aspect of the internal ring where the genital branch of the genitofemoral nerve enters the spermatic cord (Fig. 10.4). It is hazardous to apply electrocautery in this area because of the risk of injury to the nerve. Electrocautery is usually applied when raising the peritoneal flap at the beginning of the transabdominal preperitoneal operation, and the dissection should start 1 cm above the internal ring.

There is another dangerous zone inferior to the iliopubic tract and lateral to the gonadal vessels, the "triangle of pain," where one can find the genitofemoral and lateral femoral cutaneous nerves. Stapling in this area may injure either of these nerves. Together, the area between the vas deferens medially and the iliopubic tract superiorly and laterally constitutes "the square of doom," where staples or electrocautery should NEVER be applied to avoid irreversible nerve injury (Fig. 10.5).

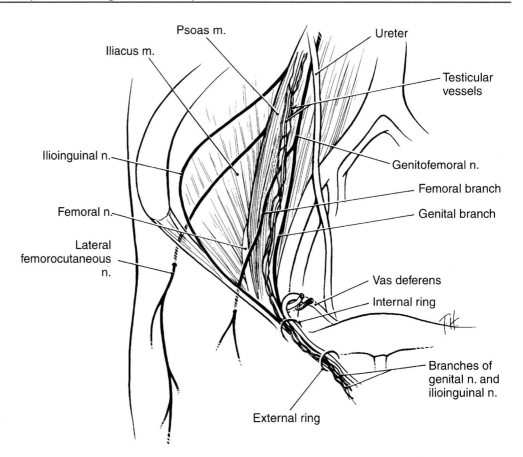

Fig. 10.4 Lateral nerves of the groin

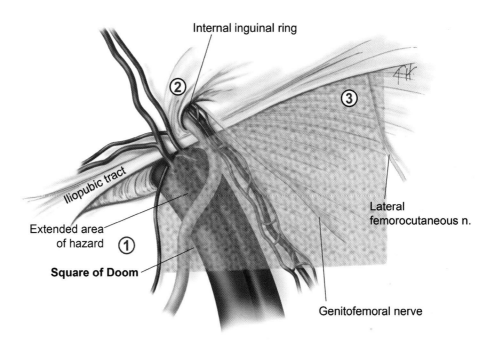

Fig. 10.5 Square of doom, delineated by the vas deferens medially and the inguinal ligament lateral and superiorly

Patient and Port Positioning

The patient is placed in the supine position with the legs together. The bladder is catheterized to prevent any obstruction of the view and to minimize the risk of injury to the bladder during dissection of the preperitoneal space.

One monitor is placed at the foot of the table. *Both arms are tucked* to allow the surgeon to stand behind the shoulder opposite to the hernia, and the camera assistant to stand on the other side of the patient. Steep Trendelenburg is required in order to remove the small bowel from the pelvic area. Three ports are necessary for this operation: a 10-mm umbilical port for the laparoscope and two 5-mm ports which can be placed at the junction of a line between umbilicus and the anterior superior iliac spine along the lateral border of the rectus muscle on either side. Alternatively, the two 5-mm ports can be placed at midline between the umbilicus and the pubic bone (Fig. 10.6a).

A 30° laparoscope is standard. Indeed, the oblique orientation of the inguinal canal makes it difficult for a right-handed surgeon to visualize small indirect hernias and the canal itself without the 30° angle.

The most difficult hernia to operate upon is a large left indirect inguinal hernia, because the huge sac and the oblique angle of the canal do not allow for an easy dissection. Following induction of the pneumoperitoneum, which is maintained at 15 mmHg, the ports are inserted as described above. The grasping forceps and electrical scissors are introduced. If the trocars are inserted too low it can be very difficult to raise the flap and maneuver the stapler device or the fibrin glue sprayer easily. If they are too high, the small bowel will be in the way. Therefore, before inserting trocars, one should ensure that the distance is adequate by indenting the abdominal wall from the outside with a finger.

Dissection of the Preperitoneal Space

The hernia sac is reduced and the peritoneal flap is incised from lateral to medial (Fig. 10.7). The incision begins over the psoas muscle laterally, extends medially 1 cm above the deep inguinal ring to avoid the genital branch of the genital femoral nerve, and ends at the medial umbilical ligament. The peritoneal flap is dissected towards the iliac vessels inferiorly and then superiorly towards the anterior abdominal wall muscles. This peritoneal flap includes the hernia sac. This is the technique for direct hernias, but with very large indirect inguino-scrotal hernias, the distal part of the sac is divided and left within the scrotum.

The preperitoneal space is then dissected. A blunt technique with the closed scissors is used to sweep tissue in each direction. This dissection of the areolar tissue can be performed with minimal hemostasis. Cooper's ligament can now be visualized: it is a white, shiny, bony structure with small veins running on its surface. One should be very careful during the dissection around these veins of the corona mortis ("crown of death"), as bleeding from them is very hard to stop. When dissection is complete, the arch of the transversus abdominous muscle, the conjoint tendon, and the iliopubic tract can be seen. The femoral nerve is present under the iliopubic tract at the lateral aspect of the dissection running deeply but this nerve is commonly not seen. In very thin patients, the lateral femoral cutaneous nerve and the genital femoral nerve may also be identified.

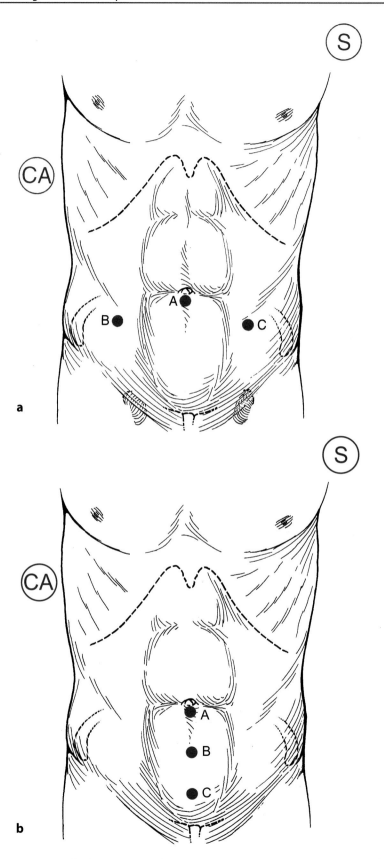

Fig. 10.6 Port positions for laparoscopic hernia repair. *S* surgeon; *CA* camera assistant. (**a**) Transabdominal preperitoneal hernia repair, and (**b**) totally extraperitoneal hernia repair. *A* umbilical telescope; *B* and *C* 5 mm trocars for the right and left hands of surgeon. *CA* camera assistant; *S* surgeon (right TEP depicted here)

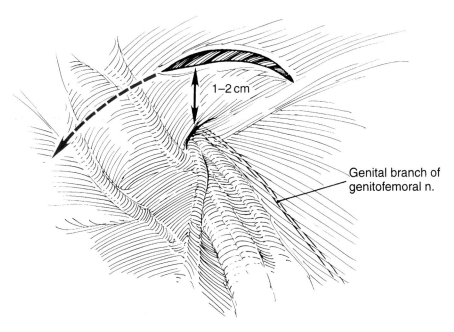

Fig. 10.7 Raising the peritoneal flap in the transabdominal preperitoneal approach

Dissection of the Cord Structures and the Vas Deferens

An important step is dissection of the spermatic cord and the vas deferens from the peritoneum, using Stoppa's parietalization technique (Figs. 10.8a, b). This will allow the spermatic cord and the vas to be completely free from the hernia sac and the peritoneum in order to lay the mesh over the hernia defect without having to cut a slit in the mesh. This dissection consists of separating the elements of the spermatic cord from the peritoneum and the peritoneal sac. It is important to continue the dissection until the peritoneum has reached the iliac vessels inferiorly. If this is not done, the mesh will need to be cut and a keyhole slot created in order to cover the hernia defects. However, on the basis of experience from the open preperitoneal hernia repair, this may predispose the repair to recurrence.

Placement of the Mesh and Fixation

When the hernia sac has been completely reduced and dissection of the preperitoneal space is completed, the mesh is introduced and fixed in place using fibrin glue (Tisseel). The mesh should be cut to an appropriate size; usually an 8 × 14-cm piece will suffice for one side, but measurements can be made using either an umbilical tape or the open jaw of the instruments themselves. The corners of the mesh should be rounded to avoid any wrinkles that might lead to a foreign body reaction, or even recurrences as described by Stoppa.

The mesh is rolled up and loaded into the umbilical port using a grasper. Once it is within the peritoneal cavity, it is unrolled into place and should cover all the hernia spaces - the aforementioned indirect, direct, and femoral spaces (Figs. 10.9 and 10.10).

Several methods can be used to place the mesh. The mesh can be marked with a sterile marker at its midline, as it is sometimes difficult to orientate it inside the small preperitoneal space. Although some surgeons are still using tacks to fix the mesh in place,

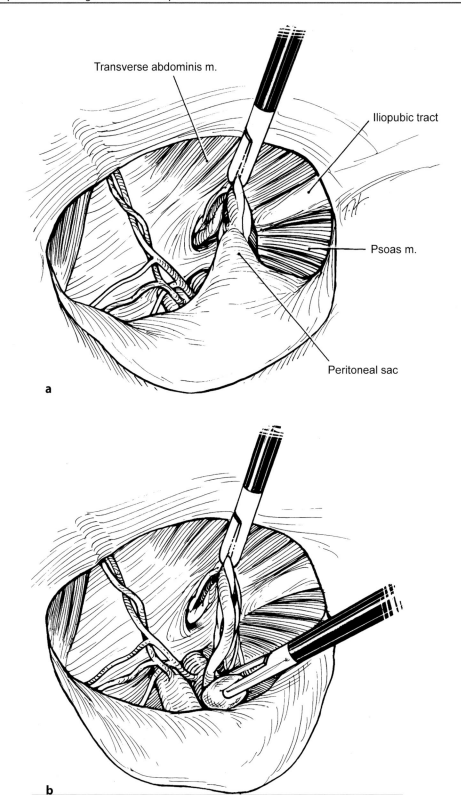

Fig. 10.8 Parietalization of the cord (STOPPA): (**a**) indirect sac before parietalization; (**b**) after parietalization

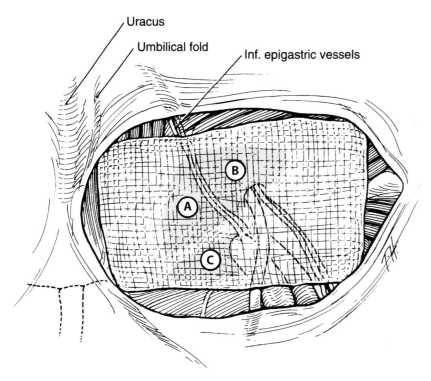

Uracus

Umbilical fold

Inf. epigastric vessels

Fig. 10.9 Mesh covering the three hernia spaces. *A* direct space; *B* indirect space; *C* femoral space

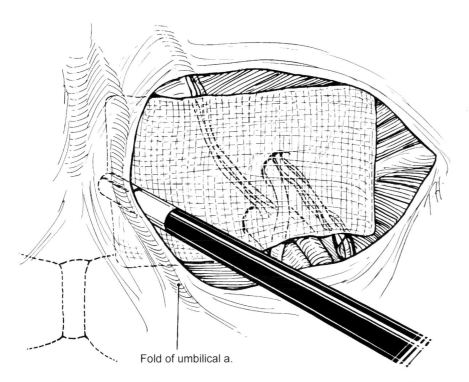

Fold of umbilical a.

Fig. 10.10 Mesh covers medially the space between the urachus and the umbilical artery

our technique of choice currently is to use fibrin glue (Tisseel) instead (Fig. 10.11). The fibrin glue is sprayed over the mesh in a thin layer, especially onto Cooper's ligament and the lateral aspect of the mesh. However, if one chooses to use tacks, the mesh fixation can begin with stapling its middle part, "three fingers" above the superior limit of the internal ring to avoid any branches of the genitofemoral nerve (Fig. 10.12). Entrapment of this

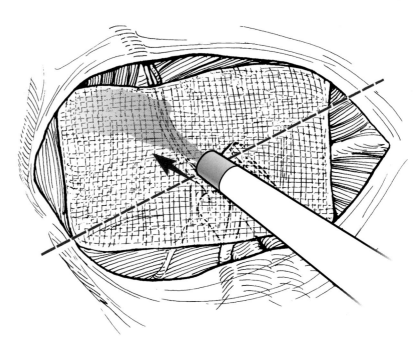

Fig. 10.11 Application of Fibrin glue (spray) for mesh fixation

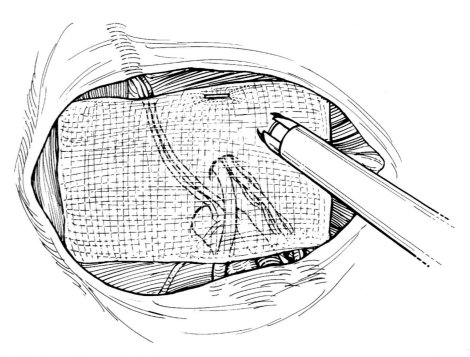

Fig. 10.12 Fixation of the mesh: the first staple

nerve can lead to severe chronic pain due to neuroma formation around the staple or tack (Fig. 10.13a, b). Then it is possible to staple both laterally and medially; laterally, it is essential to stay above the iliopubic tract, but medially staples are inserted into the rectus muscle and on Cooper's ligament.

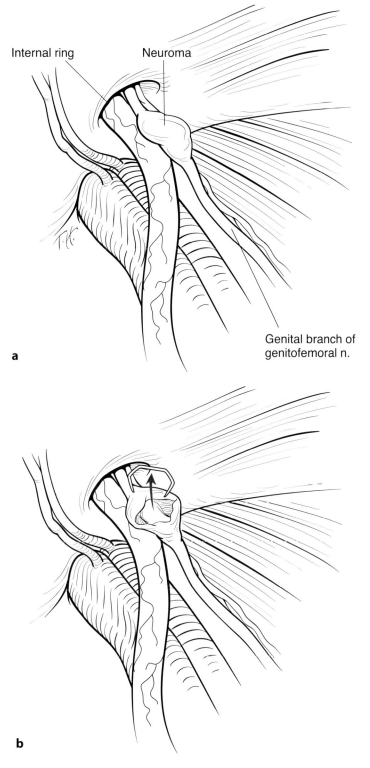

Fig. 10.13 (a, b) Neuroma formation around tacks

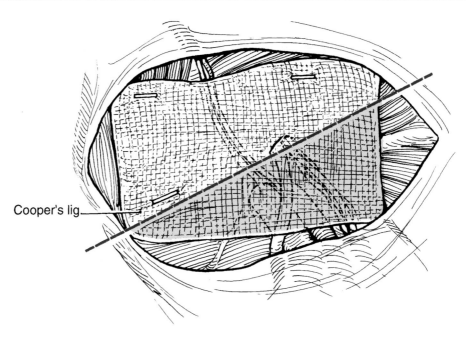

Cooper's lig

Fig. 10.14 Fixation of the mesh: showing the area in which no staples should be applied

Usually two staples are placed in Cooper's ligament and one or two in the rectus muscle. Finally, one staple laterally completes fixation of the mesh above the iliopubic tract (Fig. 10.14). Hence, a stapler with 20 staples should be sufficient for fixation of the mesh and closure of the peritoneum.

Staples or tacks are used in laparoscopic hernia repair because the mesh is smaller than that used in open surgery (as with the giant prosthesis in the Stoppa repair), so there is a slight risk of movement immediately after surgery and for perhaps 5–7 days until the inflammatory process helps to anchor the mesh.

Closure of the Peritoneum

With the mesh now secured in place, the pressure of the pneumoperitoneum is reduced to 9 mmHg. The peritoneal flap is replaced over the mesh and is closed with tacks. At this point, the tacks being used are absorbable to prevent future adhesions to the tacks. It is essential to cover the mesh completely with the flap to prevent exposure of the mesh to the underlying small bowel, thus leading to creation of adhesions and possible small bowel obstruction.

Ideally, tacking is performed in an overlap fashion (Fig. 10.15). If tacks are not available, a continuous running suture can be used to close the peritoneal flap. In order to avoid knot-tying, which might be tedious, a blocking Laparotie clip (Ethicon EndoSurgery, Cincinnati, OH) can be used to block the knot on each side (Fig. 10.16). After removal of the ports, the skin incisions are closed with single interrupted stitches after careful closure of the fascia in the 10 mm trocar port.

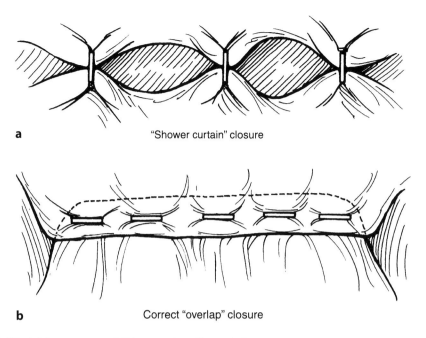

a   "Shower curtain" closure

b   Correct "overlap" closure

Fig. 10.15 (**a**) Incorrect and (**b**) correct peritoneal closures

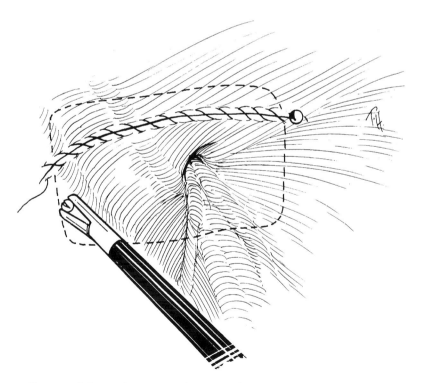

Fig. 10.16 Closure of the peritoneum using a running suture

Management of Large Indirect Hernias

For a large indirect hernia, the standard transabdominal preperitoneal hernia repair is difficult, because the sac is usually large and firmly adherent on its superior aspect to the elements of the spermatic cord; a special technique is used to overcome these difficulties.

Dissection begins with gentle and atraumatic separation of the sac from the spermatic cord structures. This is usually carried out using scissors with sharp dissection. As the sac is separated, *it is divided*, but care should always be taken to ensure that the vas is not included in the sac. It is sometimes easier to identify the vas before division of the sac commences, but usually a gradual division of the sac will allow complete separation of the sac from the cord. If oozing of blood obscures the view, the operative site should be either irrigated and aspirated or wiped with a laparoscopic 2 × 2 inch gauze. Once the peritoneal sac is completely separated from the cord, the operation proceeds as usual. The distal part of the divided sac is left open in the inguinal canal, and the proximal part of the sac is ligated using an endoloop or clips.

Totally Preperitoneal Hernia Repair (TEP)

Knowledge of the anatomy of the abdominal wall muscles, and more specifically recognition of the transition zone that occurs at the arcuate line of Douglas, is key to the success of the preperitoneal repair (Fig. 10.17).

The arcuate line of Douglas is a transitional line. Above the arcuate line, the rectus muscle has one defined anterior and posterior sheet made by aponeurotic fascia of the internal oblique and transversus abdominous muscle. Below the arcuate line, all fascial layers of the abdominal muscles lie in front of the rectus muscle, and behind the rectus muscle itself there is only the transversalis fascia. It is therefore essential to get below the arcuate line in order to start the preperitoneal dissection, which is located approximately midway between the umbilicus and the pubis (Fig. 10.18).

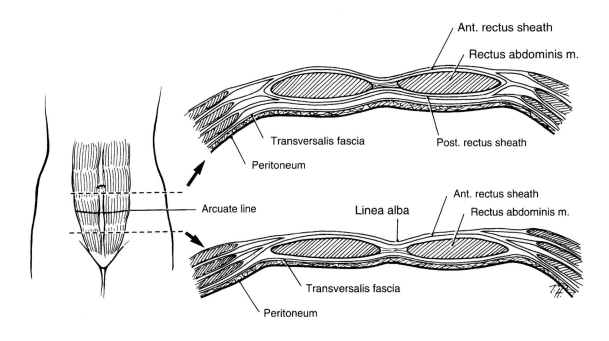

Fig. 10.17 Anatomy of the muscles of the abdominal wall

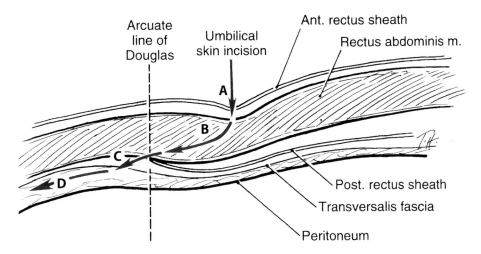

Fig. 10.18 Hernia repair: *A* division of anterior rectus sheet; *B* retraction of rectus muscle; *C* oblique dissection above posterior rectus sheet; *D* entry to the preperitoneal space

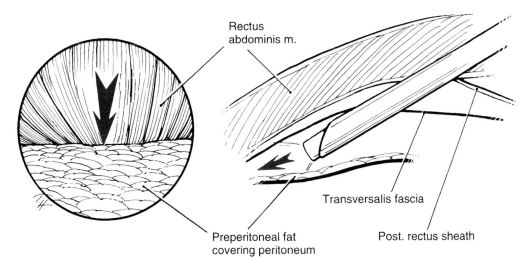

Fig. 10.19 Laparoscopic view of the preperitoneal space

The operation is started by making an incision in the umbilicus. Two retractors are used to slide the lips of the incision to the right if the hernia is located on the right side, or to the left if the hernia is located on that side. The anterior rectus sheath on the side of the hernia is then opened under direct vision, and two stay sutures of 2–0 vicryl are placed on each edge. The rectus muscle is then separated by two retractors introduced into the rectus muscle itself so that the posterior fascia can be visualized.

It is imperative at this point not to cross the posterior fascia of the rectus muscle but instead to head downwards towards the symphysis pubis in an oblique fashion using either the index finger or a small peanut with an angulation of about 30°. That will lead to the preperitoneal space below the arcuate line of Douglas (Fig. 10.19).

At this point, the preperitoneal space is dissected using a balloon spacer under direct vision with a 0° laparoscope (Fig. 10.20). While the balloon is inflated, the rectus muscle should be seen anterior and superior, and the preperitoneal fat and peritoneum

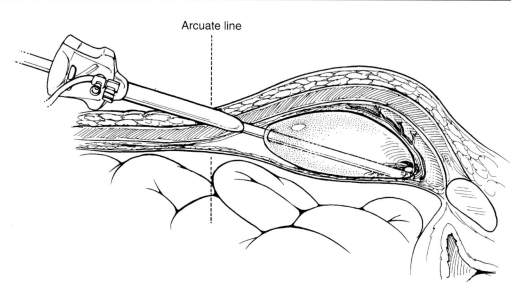

Fig. 10.20 Balloon dissection of the preperitoneal space

should be seen posterior. One should be careful to dissect in such a way that the inferior epigastric vessels stay with the rectus muscle, as otherwise they will be in the way of dissection and may need to be ligated. The balloon should stay in place for about 15 s to tamponade any bleeding. Next, the Hasson port is introduced with a video laparoscope, using the same angulation of about 30°.

Two 5-mm ports are placed at midline between the umbilicus and the symphysis pubis to operate on both sides (Fig. 10.6b). Care should be taken not to perforate the peritoneum, which will result in pneumoperitoneum and loss of space. It is obvious that the space created using this technique is small and the movements of the instruments are accordingly limited. Perforation of the peritoneum will allow CO_2 to escape into the abdominal cavity, which will subsequently compress the space and reduce it further. If this occurs, the pressures in the abdomen and the preperitoneal space must be allowed to balance before dissection continues. This is done by opening the peritoneal defect widely and inserting a Veress needle into the abdomen to allow the exit of CO_2. The perforation can be closed using an endoloop or a 5-mm clip applier.

After all ports are in place, it is imperative to proceed in the following manner: Cooper's ligament is identified medially with extreme importance placed on identification of the *fluttering of the iliac vein*. These two structures are the key anatomical landmarks in this procedure, as they will aid in defining the inferior aspect of the dissection. All dissections occur *above* this level. It is possible to injure the iliac vein, and we have seen reports of ligation of the iliac vein, which had been mistaken for a hernia sac. Once the iliac vein is identified with a careful dissection, the next step is the identification of the inferior epigastric vessels. This will delineate the internal ring and the triangle of Hasselbach. Following the internal ring medially and towards the iliac vein, one can always find the vas deferens. Once the vas deferens is dissected out, the cord structures are also separated from the sac using a soft and gentle blunt dissection. These structures are usually found behind the sac. The sac is then separated from the cord structures and vas deferens, and in this situation there are two possible scenarios. The first is a small sac that can be easily reduced.

The second is a large sac, in which case we recommend amputating the sac while paying attention to its contents and leaving the distal part of the sac open in the internal ring of the inguinal canal, and closing the proximal opening either with clips or a loop. One trick is to insert a small silk suture and tie a knot, thus effectively ligating the sac before amputating it, avoiding a loss of insufflation of the preperitoneal space and preventing pneumoperitoneum. Once the mesh is placed, we recommend using fibrin sealant (Tisseel) to fix the mesh in lieu of tackers (Fig. 10.11). This is done using an aerosol spray, attached to one of the open trocars, so there is no excessive pressure inside the abdomen. It is not important to differentiate the application of Tisseel under the mesh or above the mesh, as both will achieve the same results. It is important to always use the most lightweight large pore mesh, so as to avoid or minimize the risk of contraction of the mesh through foreign body reaction.

The operation ends by gradually removing each port, starting laterally. A grasper is left to keep the mesh in place. Finally, the last port for the camera is removed.

The obvious advantage of this technique over the transabdominal approach is that the peritoneum does not have to be closed over the mesh. The potential complications that may be associated with the transabdominal approach are avoided, as the peritoneum is not entered.

Selected Further Reading

Avery C, Foley RJ, Prasad A (1995) Simplifying mesh placement during laparoscopic hernia repair. Br J Surg 82(5):642

Avital S, Werbin N (1997) Conventional versus laparoscopic surgery for inguinal-hernia repair. N Engl J Med 337(15):1089–1090

Banerjee AK (1995) Laparoscopic alternatives for the repair of inguinal hernias. Ann Surg 222(2):213–214

Barkun IS, Wexler MJ, Hinchey EJ, Thibeault D, Meakins JL (1995) Laparoscopic versus open inguinal herniorrhaphy: preliminary results of a randomized controlled trial. Surgery 118(4):703–709

Brooks DC (1994) A prospective comparison of laparoscopic and tension-free open herniorrhaphy. Arch Surg 129(4):361–366

Cornell RB, Kerlakian GM (1994) Early complications and outcomes of the current technique of transperitoneal laparoscopic herniorrhaphy and a comparison to the traditional open approach. Am J Surg 168(3):275–279

Dahlstrand U, Wollert S, Nordin P, Sandblom G, Gunnarsson U (2009) Emergency femoral hernia repair: a study based on a national register. Ann Surg 249(4):672–676

Deans GT, Wilson MS, Royston CM, Brough WA (1995) Recurrent inguinal hernia after laparoscopic repair: possible cause and prevention. Br J Surg 82(4):539–541

Evans MD, Williams GL, Stephenson BM (2009) Low recurrence rate after laparoscopic (TEP) and open (Lichtenstein) inguinal hernia repair: a randomized, multicenter trial with 5-year follow-up. Ann Surg 250(2):354–355

Fitzgibbons RI Jr, Salerno GM, Filipi CJ, Hunter WJ, Watson P (1994) A laparoscopic intraperitoneal onlay mesh technique for the repair of an indirect inguinal hernia. Ann Surg 219(2):144–156

Fitzgibbons RJ Jr, Camps I, Cornet DA et al (1995a) Laparoscopic inguinal herniorrhaphy. Results of a multicenter trial. Ann Surg 221(1):3–13

Fitzgibbons R, Katkhouda N, McKernan JB, Steffes B et al (1995b) Laparoscopic Inguinal Herniorraphy, results of a Multicentric trial. Ann Surg 221:3–13

Fujita T (2009) Laparoscopic versus open mesh repair for inguinal hernia. Ann Surg 250(2):353–354

Geraghty JG, Grace PA, Quereshi A, Bouchier-Hayes D, Osborne DH (1994) Simple new technique for laparoscopic inguinal hernia repair. Br J Surg 81(1):93

Hallén M, Bergenfelz A, Westerdahl J (2008) Laparoscopic extraperitoneal inguinal hernia repair versus open mesh repair: long-term follow-up of a randomized controlled trial. Surgery 143(3):313–317

Hetz SP, Holcomb JB (1996) Combined laparoscopic exploration and repair of inguinal hernias. J Am Colt Surg 182(4):364–366

Horgan LF, Shelton JC, ORiordan DC, Moore DP, Winslet MC, Davidson BR (1996) Strengths and weaknesses of laparoscopic and open mesh inguinal hernia repair: a randomized controlled experimental study. Br J Surg 83(10):1463–1467

Jacobs DO (2004) Mesh repair of inguinal hernias–redux. N Engl J Med 350(18): 1895–1897

Kald A, Smedh K, Anderberg B (1995) Laparoscopic groin hernia repair: results of 200 consecutive herniorraphies. Br J Surg 82(5):618–620

Katkhouda N, Mouiel J (1992) Laparoscopic Treatment of Inguinal Hernia of the Adult. Chirugie Endoscopique 3:7–10

Katkhouda N, Mouiel J (1993) Laparoscopic treatment of inguinal hernia. A personal approach. Endosc Surg New Technol 1:193–197

Katkhouda N, Campos GMR, Mavor E, Trussler A, Khalil M, Stoppa R (1999) Laparoscopic extraperitoneal inguinal hernia repair. A safe approach based on the understanding of the anatomy of the rectus sheath. Surg Endosc 13:1243–1246

Katkhouda N, Mavor E, Friedlander MH, Mason RJ, Kiyabu M, Grant SW, Achanta K, Kirkman EL, Narayanan K, Essani R (2001) Use of fibrin sealant for prosthetic mesh fixation in laparoscopic extraperitoneal inguinal hernia repair. Ann Surg 233(1):18–25

Kouhia ST, Huttunen R, Silvasti SO, Heiskanen JT, Ahtola H, Uotila-Nieminen M, Kiviniemi VV, Hakala T (2009) Lichtenstein hernioplasty versus totally extraperitoneal laparoscopic hernioplasty in treatment of recurrent inguinal hernia–a prospective randomized trial. Ann Surg 249(3):384–387

Kozol R, Lange PM, Kosir M et al (1997) A prospective, randomized study of open vs laparoscopic inguinal hernia repair. An assessment of postoperative pain. Arch Surg 132(3):292–295

Lawrence K, McWhinnie D, Goodwin A et al (1995) Randomized controlled trial of laparoscopic versus open repair of inguinal hernia: early results. Br Med J 311(7011): 981–985

Liem MS, Kallewaard JW, de Smet AM, van Vroonhoven TJ (1995) Does hypercarbia develop faster during laparoscopic herniorrhaphy than during laparoscopic cholecystectomy? Assessment with continuous blood gas monitoring. Anes Analg 81(6): 1243–1249

Liem MS, van der Graaf CJ (1997) Comparison of conventional anterior surgery and laparo scopic surgery for inguinal hernia repair. N Engl J Med 336(22):1541–1547

Liem MS, van der Graaf Y, Zwart RC, Geurts I, van Vroonhoven TJ (1997) A randomized comparison of physical performance following laparoscopic and open inguinal hernia repair. The Coala Trial Group. Br J Surg 84(1):64–67

Liem MS, van Steensel CJ, Boelhouwer RU et al (1996) The learning curve for totally extraperitoneal laparoscopic inguinal hernia repair. Am J Surg 171(2):281–285

Liem MS, van Vroonhoven TJ (1996) Laparoscopic inguinal hernia repair. Br J Surg 83(9):1197–1204

Lowham AS, Filipi CJ, Fitzgibbons RJ Jr et al (1997) Mechanisms of hernia recurrence after peritoneal mesh repair. Traditional and laparoscopic. Ann Surg 225(4):422–431

Memon MA, Rice D, Donohue JH (1997) Laparoscopic herniorrhaphy. J Am Coil Surg 184(3):325–335

Moreno-Egea A, Torralba Martínez JA, Morales Cuenca G, Aguayo Albasini JL (2004) Randomized clinical trial of fixation vs nonfixation of mesh in total extraperitoneal inguinal hernioplasty. Arch Surg 139(12):1376–1379

Neumayer L, Giobbie-Hurder A, Jonasson O, Fitzgibbons R Jr, Dunlop D, Gibbs J, Reda D, Henderson W; Veterans Affairs Cooperative Studies Program 456 Investigators (2004) Open mesh versus laparoscopic mesh repair of inguinal hernia. N Engl J Med 29;350(18):1819–1827

Novik B (2005) Randomized trial of fixation vs nonfixation of mesh in total extraperitoneal inguinal hernioplasty. Arch Surg 140(8):811–812

Oka M, Hiwaki K, Takao K, Iizuka N, Yamamoto K, Suzuki T (1996) The saline ballooning method for peritoneal dissection during laparoscopic herniorrhaphy. Arch Surg 131(4):448–449

Olmi S, Scaini A, Erba L, Guaglio M, Croce E (2007) Quantification of pain in laparoscopic transabdominal preperitoneal (TAPP) inguinal hernioplasty identifies marked differences between prosthesis fixation systems. Surgery 142(1):40–46

Panton ON, Panton RJ (1994) Laparoscopic hernia repair. Am J Surg 167(5):535–537

Payne JH Jr, Grininger LM, Izawa MT, Podoll EF, Lindahl PT, Balfour J (1994) Laparoscopic or open inguinal herniorrhaphy? A randomized prospective trial. Arch Surg 129(9): 973–979

Sampath P, Yeo CT, Campbell TN (1995) Nerve injury associated with laparoscopic inguinal herniorrhaphy. Surgery 118(5):829–833

Sandbilcher P, Draxl H, Gstir H et al (1996) Laparoscopic repair of recurrent inguinal hernias. Am J Surg 171(3):366–368

Stoker DL, Speigelhalter DJ, Singh R, Wellwood JM (1994) Laparoscopic versus open inguinal hernia repair: randomized prospective trial. Lancet 343(8908):1243–1245

Swanstrom LL (1996) Laparoscopic herniorrhaphy. Surg Clin N Am 76(3):483–491

Vogt DM, Curet MJ, Pitcher DE, Martin DT, Zucker KA (1995) Preliminary results of a prospective randomized trial of laparoscopic onlay versus conventional inguinal herniorrhaphy. Am J Surg 169(1):84–89

Wilson MS, Deans GT, Brough WA (1995) Prospective trial comparing Lichtenstein with laparoscopic tension-free mesh repair of inguinal hernia. Br J Surg 82(2):274–277

Incisional and Ventral Hernia Repair Including Component Separation

11

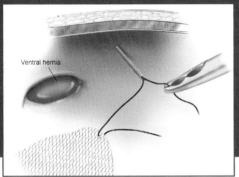

Indications

Ventral and incisional hernias centered around the umbilicus and on or close to the midline are good indications for the laparoscopic approach. Lateral hernias close to bony structures (ribs, pubis, iliac crest) or following incisions on the flank are difficult and require special techniques (Fig. 11.1).

Technique

Positioning

The patient should be in the supine position on the operating room table with both arms tucked. This will give the surgeon and assistant/camera holder sufficient room to stand on the same side. If the hernia being repaired is in the lower abdomen, a Foley catheter should be placed to prevent bladder injury. The operating room table should be capable of rotating in different directions to help with exposure of the hernia and to use gravity to assist in manipulating the bowel away from the operative field.

N. Katkhouda, *Advanced Laparoscopic Surgery*,
DOI: 10.1007/978-3-540-74843-4_11, © Springer-Verlag Berlin Heidelberg 2011

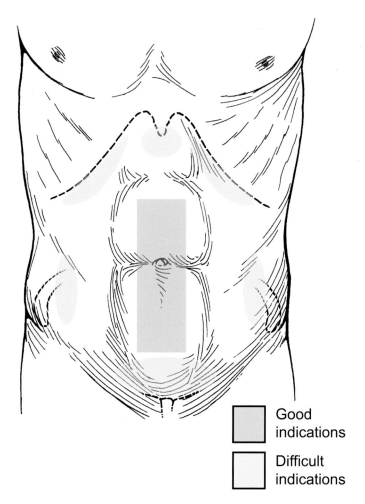

Good indications

Difficult indications

Fig. 11.1 Indications for laparoscopic ventral hernia repair. *Orange color* on the middle indicates sites of good indication for laparoscopic ventral or incisional hernia repairs. *Yellow color* on the periphery indicates sites of less favorable indications for laparoscopic ventral and incisional hernia repairs

Pneumoperitoneum

Pneumoperitoneum can be achieved with either the Hasson technique or by using the Veress needle. This can be done in the midline if it is not close to the hernia, but if the hernia is in the midline, Palmers point in front of 11th rib on the left side is a safe place. If there are any doubts about Veress needle placement, the Hasson technique should be used.

Port Placement

Usually, three ports placed in a triangulated fashion suffice for a ventral hernia repair. The ports should be placed on the opposite side of the hernia. For example, if the hernia is from an open appendectomy, the ports should be placed on the left side of the patient. For midline hernias, the ports can be placed on either side, but it is safer to place them on the opposite side of a previous surgical site to decrease the risk of getting into

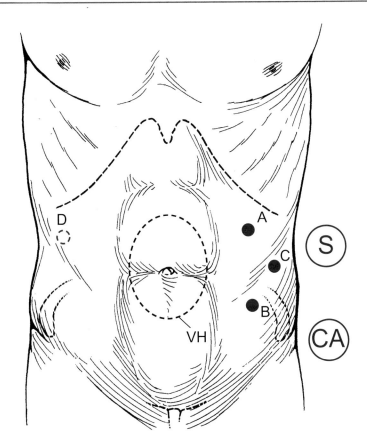

Fig. 11.2 Trocar placement for laparoscopic incisional hernia repair. *Dotted line* indicates incisional or ventral hernia. *C* camera; *B* left hand of surgeron; *A* right hand of surgeon; *D* additional 5 mm trocar for tacker. *S* surgeon; *CA* camera assistant

adhesions (Fig. 11.2). For example, if a midline hernia is from an open left hemicolectomy, it is better to place the ports on the right side of the abdomen. One port should be at least 10 mm in order to introduce the mesh into the abdominal cavity. The additional trocars for the introduction of the tacker are 5 mm.

Adhesiolysis

The first step is to reduce the hernia contents and free up the abdominal wall from adhesions. Adhesiolysis should be done with either sharp dissection with scissors or with the harmonic scalpel (Fig. 11.3). Using cautery with scissors can be very dangerous, as it can result in an unnoticed bowel injury and should be done very carefully. After the adhesions are taken down, the contents of the hernia should be reduced into the abdominal cavity by traction from inside the abdominal cavity and with the help of the assistant from outside the abdominal cavity to push them into the abdomen. If the hernia sac contains only omentum, it can be amputated, reduced, and then removed from the abdominal cavity.

The hernia can be excised and removed. This will decrease the risk of seroma, but if it is very close to skin, it may result in devascularization of the skin or a puncture hole in the skin.

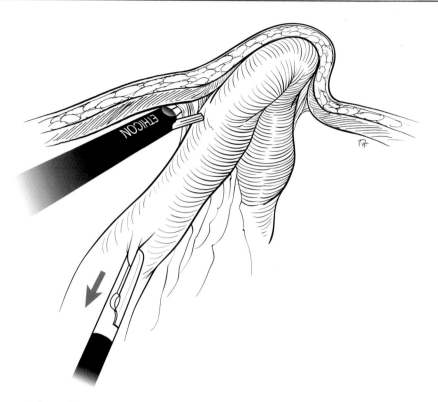

Fig. 11.3 Adhesiolysis using the harmonic shears

Measurement of the Hernia Defect

The hernia defect can be measured from the inside or the outside of the abdomen (Fig. 11.4). The measurement from inside is more precise and is performed using a paper ruler introduced into the abdominal cavity, or using a suture stretched across the hernia defect with two graspers and measured outside.

A thin long spinal needle is used to measure the defect from the outside of the abdominal cavity. The needle is pushed through the skin to exit superiorly, inferiorly, and on the right and left side of the hernia, right 5 cm away from the edge of the fascial defect so as to mark the defect and the 5 cm overlap (Fig. 11.5). These four points are marked and drawn on the skin to measure the defect. It is important to remember that as the inside girth of abdominal cavity is shorter than the outside girth, this technique tends to overestimate the hernia defect size and should be considered when the transfascial sutures are passed through the abdominal wall. *Deflating the abdomen at this point* decreases the difference between the inside and outside girth (larger diameter), making the measurement from the outside more precise.

Placement of Mesh

Bilayer mesh, with one side made of materials that do not adhere to the bowel and the other side made of materials that facilitate tissue ingrowth in contact with fascia and muscles, should always be used for ventral hernia repair. It is very important to make sure that the side of the mesh that touches on the bowel side stays on the correct side.

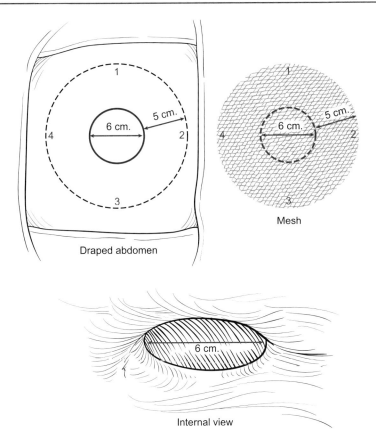

Fig. 11.4 Measurement of the hernia defect (6 cm in this example) with a 5-cm overlap. *1, 2, 3, 4* indicate the periphery of the mesh and the site of introduction of the suture passer

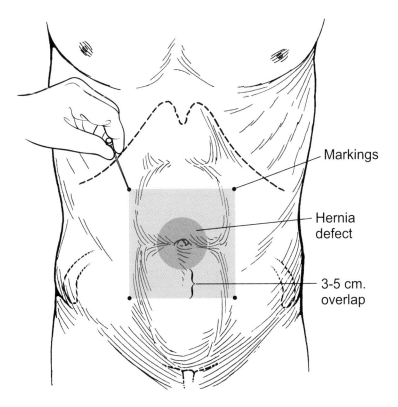

Fig. 11.5 Technique using the 20 gauge or spinal needle to mark the hernia defect and 5 cm overlap

A minimum of 3–5 cm of overlap on each edge is necessary to decrease the risk of recurrence. For example, if the hernia defect is 5 × 5 cm, the mesh should be between 11 × 11 and 15 × 15 cm. The mesh is rolled and introduced through the 10 mm port. Adding a 5-mm port on the other side of the abdomen can help with pulling the mesh inside and later the port can also be used to place tacks (Fig. 11.2). The following are two techniques that can be used to fix the mesh to the abdominal wall:

1. *Double Crown technique*: In this technique, the mesh is fixed to the abdominal wall with two rows of tacks. The first row is placed right at the fascial defect and the second row is placed at the edge of mesh approximately 6–10 mm from the edge. We now use the absorbable tacks that will dissolve in less than 6 months (Fig. 11.6).
2. *Transfacial sutures*: In this technique, four nonabsorbable sutures are placed at each corner of the mesh (Fig. 11.7). These sutures are tied twice and then cut long enough to be passed through the abdominal wall. The length of overlap is added to each side of the hernia mark on the skin and a new marking that corresponds to the mesh size is drawn on the skin. The exit site of these sutures is then marked on the skin. After the mesh is introduced into the abdominal cavity, these four sutures are passed through the abdominal wall. The suture passer is introduced through the abdominal wall through a stab wound (Fig. 11.8). The mesh should be flat, but not under too much tension. The transfascial sutures are then tied (Fig. 11.9). The dimple in the skin can be fixed easily by pulling the skin away from the abdominal wall. Tacks are then placed at the edge of the mesh as needed to decrease the risk of bowel herniation between the mesh and the abdominal wall. The addition of a 5-mm port on the opposite side, if not previously placed, will help in placing tacks on the side that is close to the ports.

At the end, Tisseel can be sprayed on the tacks and the edge of the mesh, which may help in decreasing adhesion of the bowel to the tacks; spraying Tisseel between the mesh and the fascia may also help reduce the risk of seroma formation (Fig. 11.10).

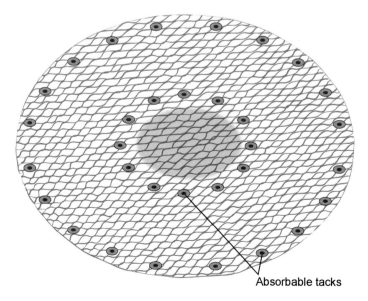

Absorbable tacks

Fig. 11.6 "Double crown" fixation technique using absorbable tacks

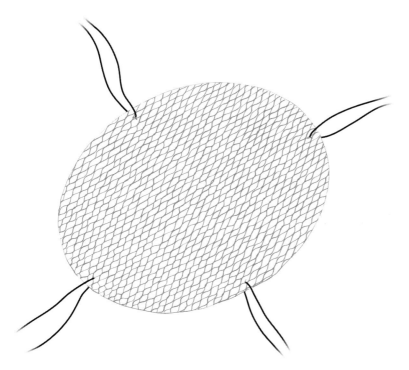

Fig. 11.7 Transfascial sutures for fixation of mesh

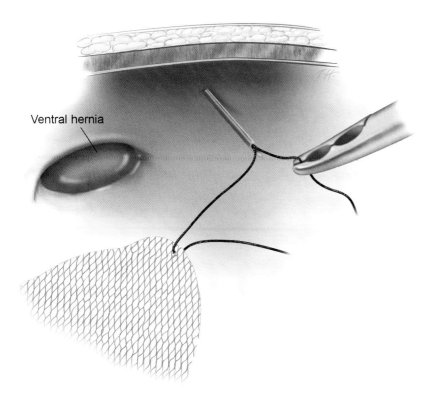

Ventral hernia

Fig. 11.8 Passage of the suture passer for transfascial fixation of the mesh

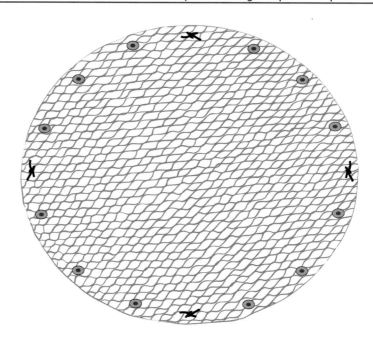

Fig. 11.9   Completion of the "suture and tack" technique

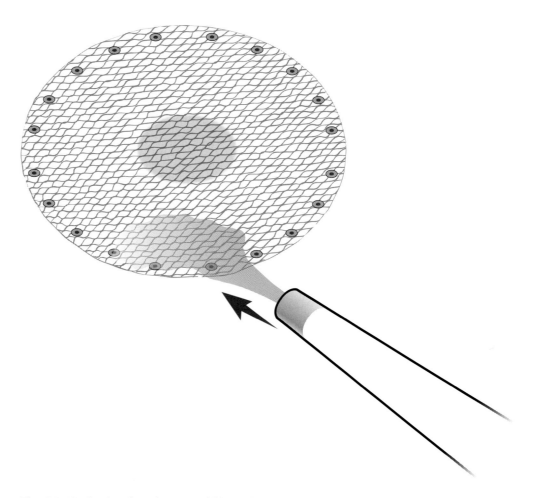

Fig. 11.10   Optional application of fibrin glue on the tacks to reduce the risk of small bowel adhesions

Difficult Ventral or Incisional Hernias

Incisional or ventral hernias close to bony structures (the xyphoid process, ribs, pubis, pelvis) or following flank incisions for nephrectomy or spine surgery are very difficult to fix. (Fig. 11.1).

For the hernia around the xyphoid process or the ribs, one has to take down the falciform ligament and place the mesh above the liver. The anchoring of the mesh should use tacks or intracoporeal sutures, *without* use of a suture passer.

For suprapubic hernias, the inferior border of the mesh should be fixed with tacks to the pubic bone and to Cooper's ligament.

Finally, hernias of the flank can possibly be more challenging, as they do not present as hernias but rather as eventrations due to muscular nerve atrophy. The author prefers an open approach for larger hernias.

Pain Following Laparoscopic Ventral or Incisional Hernia Repair

The disposition of the intercostal nerves shows that some minor injury to the nerves is unavoidable, especially with the suture and tack repair (Fig. 11.11). The sutures will sometimes entrap a nerve, resulting in chronic pain. The patient should be forewarned about the occurrence of postoperative pain during the preoperative clinic visit. Local injections are used, and sometimes removal of the responsible suture with the inherent neuroma is the last resort.

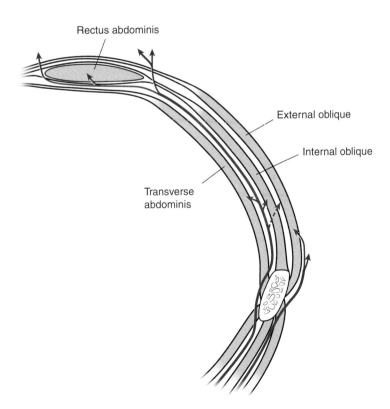

Fig. 11.11 Disposition of the intercostal nerves as they innervate the muscles of the abdominal wall; this may explain postsurgical chronic pain issues

Laparoscopic Component Separation

The goal is to divide laparoscopically the fascia of the external oblique laterally to the rectus sheath. This will separate the components of the large muscles of the abdomen and reduce the size of the midline defect and consequently, the size of the mesh to be used. It will also reduce the tension on the closure of the defect.

Three trocars are placed, one 10 mm under the costal margin, another 10 mm in the flank, and a final 5 mm trocar in the right lower quadrant (Fig. 11.12). The Hasson technique is used for the right upper quadrant port (A); the aponeurosis of the external oblique is identified and opened, and a balloon dissector is inflated *beneath the external oblique and above the internal oblique* to create a working space(Fig. 11.13). A 10-mm trocar (B) in the flank is inserted into the space to allow for an electrical scissor to divide the fascia of the external oblique laparoscopically, just lateral to the rectus sheath going downwards towards the right lower quadrant (Fig. 11.14). In order to divide the upper part of the external oblique fascia, a 5-mm trocar is inserted (C). The camera is moved from the right upper quadrant trocar to the middle 10 mm trocar, and a scissor is introduced into the 5 mm trocar to complete the division. The same maneuver is performed on the opposite side.

After the component separation is finished, it is possible to perform an incisional hernia repair using a *smaller* mesh, as the component separation allows the edges of the fascial defect to be brought closer together; alternatively, a full laparoscopic incisional hernia repair with a sublay mesh can be performed.

The main advantage of the laparoscopic component separation technique is to avoid the risk of devascularizing the skin, which can occur with the open method.

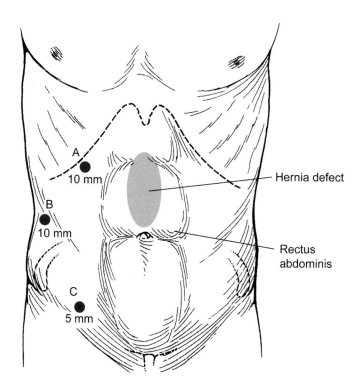

Fig. 11.12 Trocar placement for laparoscopic component separation. *A* initial introduction site for the balloon dissector, and the Hasson trocar for the camera; *B* trocar port for the electrical scissors; *C* additional 5 mm port for the scissor to finish up the division of the cephalad portion of the external oblique fascia

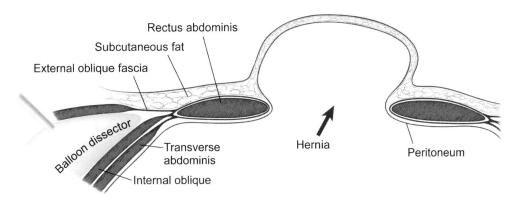

Fig. 11.13 Introduction of the balloon dissection in the space beneath the fascia of the external oblique and above the internal oblique

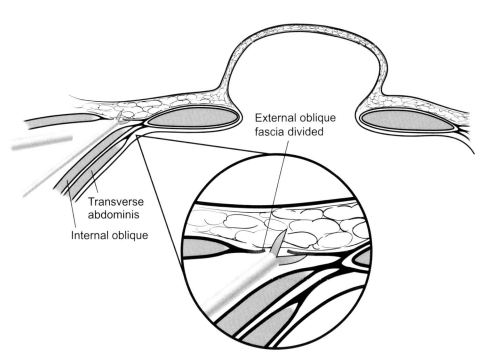

Fig. 11.14 Division of the external oblique fascia with electrical scissors, until the subcutaneous fat is visible. This will achieve a separation of the components and a subsequent release of the tension on the closure of the defect

Selected Further Reading

Alvarez C (2004) Open mesh versus laparoscopic mesh hernia repair. N Engl J Med 351(14):1463–1465

Bingener J, Buck L, Richards M, Michalek J, Schwesinger W, Sirinek K (2007) Long-term outcomes in laparoscopic vs open ventral hernia repair. Arch Surg 142(6):562–567

Fujita F, Lahmann B, Otsuka K, Lyass S, Hiatt JR, Phillips EH (2004) Quantification of pain and satisfaction following laparoscopic and open hernia repair. Arch Surg 139(6):596–600

Kennealey PT, Johnson CS, Tector AJ 3rd, Selzer DJ (2009) Laparoscopic incisional hernia repair after solid-organ transplantation. Arch Surg 144(3):228–233

Malas M, Katkhouda N (2002) Herniation through the falciform ligament following laparoscopic surgery. Surg Laparosc Endosc 12:115–116

Novitsky YW, Cobb WS, Kercher KW, Matthews BD, Sing RF, Heniford BT (2006) Laparoscopic ventral hernia repair in obese patients: a new standard of care. Arch Surg 141(1):57–61

Ponsky TA, Nam A, Orkin BA, Lin PP (2006) Open, intraperitoneal, ventral hernia repair: lessons learned from laparoscopy. Arch Surg 141(3):304–306

Splenectomy (Total and Partial) and Splenopancreatectomy 12

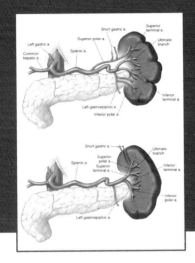

Preoperative Requirements and Workup

Classic Laparoscopic Splenectomy

Laparoscopic splenectomy is a difficult procedure that should only be performed by an experienced laparoscopic surgeon or under the direct supervision of such a surgeon. As always, the entire team should be adequately prepared.

The surgeon should check the instrument set personally to ensure that everything is available, specifically clip appliers, atraumatic graspers, liver fan retractors, and an irrigation suction machine with the capacity for hydrodissection. An open tray with a number 10 or 20 blade should be immediately available in case there is a need for conversion. Harmonic shears (Ethicon Endosurgery Inc.) are especially useful because they can reduce the number of clips used during division of the short gastric vessels, and can also function as a grasper.

It is essential that patients presenting with idiopathic thrombocytopenic purpura (ITP) are worked up appropriately by the referring hematologists. The anesthesiologist must make sure that there is a suitable blood and platelet supply in the operating room prior to the start of the procedure. An orogastric tube is placed to decompress the stomach.

The patient should be vaccinated against pneumococcus, *H. influenza* and menningococcus (triple vaccine) at least 2 weeks prior to surgery.

N. Katkhouda, *Advanced Laparoscopic Surgery*,
DOI: 10.1007/978-3-540-74843-4_12, © Springer-Verlag Berlin Heidelberg 2011

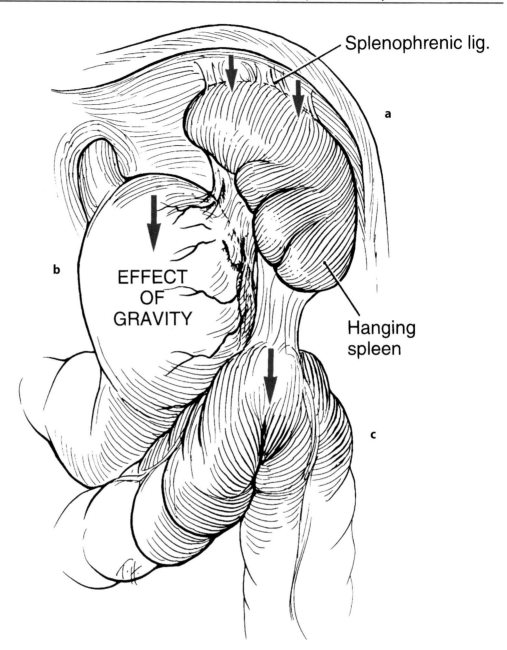

Fig. 12.3 Effects of reverse Trendelenburg and 60° elevation: (**a**) splenic pedicle put under tension; (**b**) stomach falls down; (**c**) splenic flexure put under strain

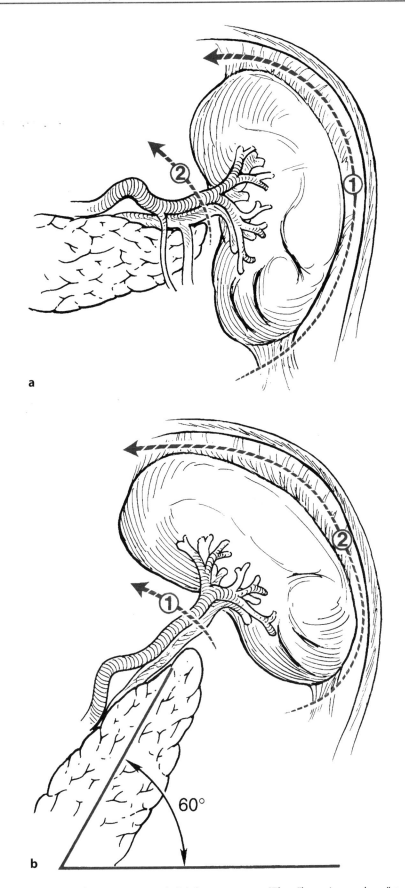

Fig. 12.4 (**a**) Open splenectomy, and (**b**) laparoscopy (The "hanging spleen" technique). Numbers depict stages of the operation

Port Placement

Four to five 12 mm ports are needed for this operation (Fig. 12.5). Following insufflation using a Veress needle, the first trocar is inserted in the left upper quadrant approximately five finger-breadths below the costal margin, moving the camera closer to the spleen. This will permit full exploration of the abdominal cavity to check for the presence of accessory spleens and other intra-abdominal lesions that might require laparoscopic management.

One port is inserted on each side of the umbilical port in a triangulated manner, for the right and left hands of the surgeon. Another trocar is inserted laterally under the left costal margin for the first assistant. An optional subxiphoid trocar can be inserted for an irrigation/suction device or for a fan retractor used by the camera assistant if needed.

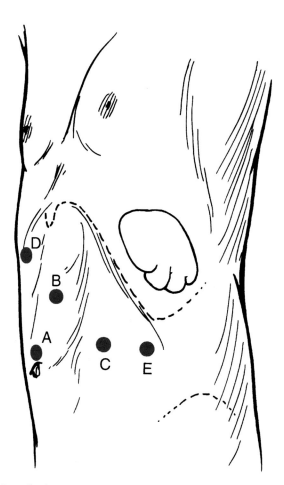

Fig. 12.5 Port positions for laparoscopic splenectomy: *A* umbilical telescope; *B* surgeon's left hand; *C* surgeon's right hand; *D* subxiphoid port for irrigation/suction or an assistant's grasper; *E* first assistant's grasper

Surgical Anatomy

Vascularization of the spleen may be of the distributed type (Fig. 12.6a) or the non-branching variant (Fig. 12.6b). Knowledge of the patient's vascular anatomy will help decide on the most appropriate dissection technique. The terminal branches of the splenic artery are depicted in Fig. 12.7. Knowledge of the anatomy of the spleen is critical, and two special features are of interest. First, as a rule, notched spleens and those with prominences have more entering arteries than those with smooth borders (usually distributed type). Second, the tail of the pancreas lies close to the hilum of the spleen and is in direct contact with the spleen in about 30% of cases, and within 1 cm of the spleen in 40%. Caution is therefore recommended before firing a linear cutter across the hilar vessels.

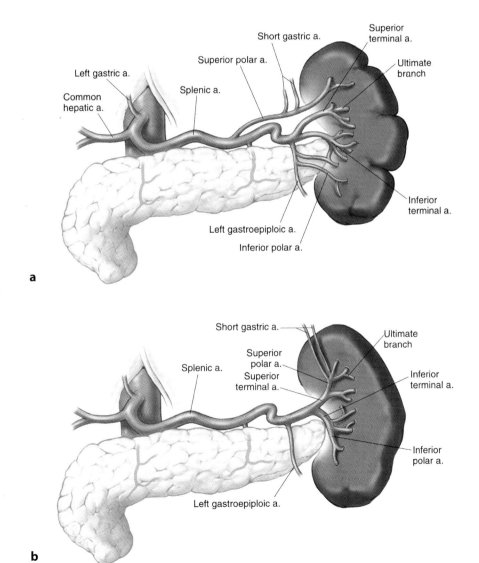

Fig. 12.6 Vascularization of the spleen: (**a**) *distributed* type with multiple splenic notches, and (**b**) *magistral* type with few splenic notches

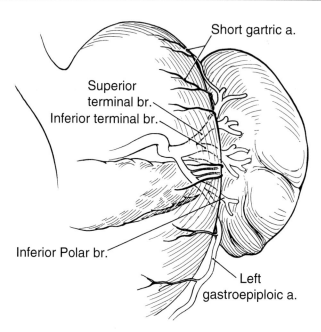

Fig. 12.7 Terminal branches of the splenic artery

Surgical Principles

■ **Anterior Approach.** The procedure follows these key steps:

- Division of the short gastric vessels and opening the lesser sac (Fig. 12.8).
- Exposure of the tail of the pancreas.
- Division of the splenocolic ligament.
- Lateral and superior retraction of the inferior pole of the spleen and division of the inferior pole vessels.
- Division of the hilar vessels.
- Division of the phrenic attachments.
- Extraction of the spleen in a bag.

■ **Technique**

Division of the Short Gastric Vessels and Exposure of the Tail of the Pancreas

The first step is division of the short gastric vessels and entry into the lesser sac along the greater curvature of the stomach. This proceeds as for a Nissen fundoplication with the exception that the dissection is carried out much closer to the spleen than to the stomach (Chap. 5). The first assistant gently grasps the fatty tissue surrounding the short gastric vessels and retracts it superiorly, while the surgeon gently retracts the stomach to the right. This will expose the short gastric vessels, which are subsequently controlled with the harmonic shears. Clips can be added for larger vessels if needed. The division is then continued superiorly and then inferiorly until the tail of the pancreas is completely exposed (Fig. 12.9).

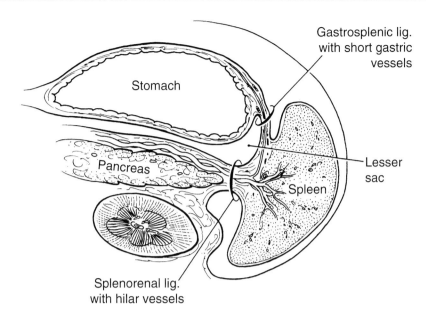

Fig. 12.8 Access to the hilar vessels through the lesser sac. Figure depicts ligaments of the posterior mesogastrum

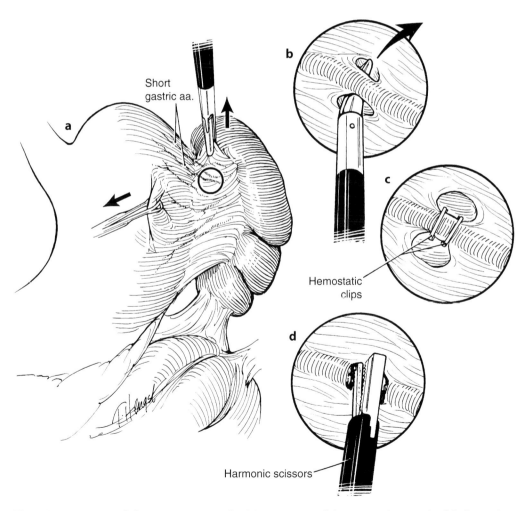

Fig. 12.9 Division of short gastric vessels: (**a**) exposure of short gastric vessels; (**b**) dissection with scissors; (**c**) clips; (**d**) harmonic shears

Exposure of the Inferior Pole of the Spleen and Division of the Inferior Pole Vessels

The next step is exposure of the inferior pole of the spleen (Fig. 12.10). The first assistant retracts the spleen superiorly and laterally with a closed Babcock clamp to expose the splenic flexure of the colon. The surgeon's left hand retracts the transverse colon inferiorly, exposing the splenocolic ligament. The ligament is divided using the harmonic shears to allow safe dissection of the inferior pole of the spleen. Once the splenocolic ligament has been divided, lateral and superior retraction will expose the inferior pole vessels that branch from the main splenic vessels. The inferior pole vessels are divided at this point, permitting full mobilization of the inferior pole of the spleen. These vessels are usually large in size and should be clipped or divided using an endo-GIA with a white load. We do not recommend the use of the harmonic shears on these vessels, as it will not achieve efficient hemostasis. Uncontrollable bleeding from these vessels can result in an early conversion to open surgery.

Division of the Hilar Vessels and Phrenic Attachments

In order to expose the hilar vessels, opposing retraction by the first assistant and the surgeon is required. The first assistant retracts the mobilized inferior pole of the spleen superiorly and laterally. The surgeon gently pushes the exposed tail of the pancreas down, creating access to the hilum and the main splenic vessels (Fig. 12.11). Division of the hilar artery and vein is a critical step that should be performed meticulously and carefully to avoid any bleeding. Use of a blunt right-angled dissector is safe.

The surgeon has two choices for ligation of the splenic vessels at the hilum of the spleen: transection of the vessels with one firing of a 30-mm Endolinear cutter using vascular staples (Fig. 12.12a), or a more formal division of the artery and vein separately between clips (Fig. 12.12b). Using a combination of clips and staplers should also be done very cautiously, as clips can result in misfiring of the stapler and subsequent bleeding from a partially divided vessel.

Finally, the attachments of the spleen to the diaphragm are divided, allowing full mobilization of the spleen.

Extraction of the Spleen in a Bag

The next step is introduction of the retrieval bag. A good trick is to push the bag to the diaphragm with the opening of the bag facing the surgeon. This will allow introduction of the spleen into the bag using a "surfing" technique. The spleen is grabbed by its attachments and rolled onto its back, using hilar and fatty attachments as a handle. Thus, the spleen is shoved in a gentle sliding motion into the bag (Fig. 12.13).

The bag is closed and the umbilical port removed. The fascia of the umbilical port can be slightly enlarged to allow extraction of the bag. The introduction of two fingers (or a Kelly clamp) to squeeze the spleen between the fingers and the anterior abdominal wall will enable morcellation of the spleen and extraction of both the bag and the splenic fragments. One should be careful not to drop any fragments in the abdomen, which can lead to splenosis and recurrent disease.

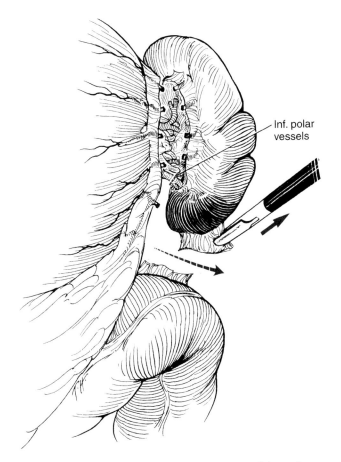

Inf. polar
vessels

Fig. 12.10 Division of the splenocolic ligament, and division of the inferior polar vessels

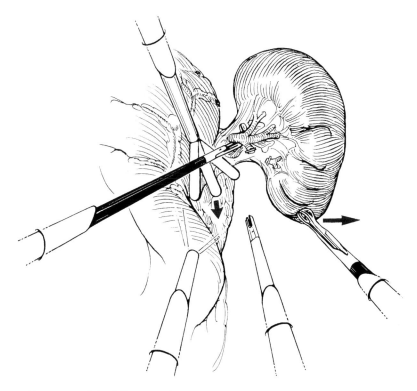

Fig. 12.11 Exposure of the hilar vessels

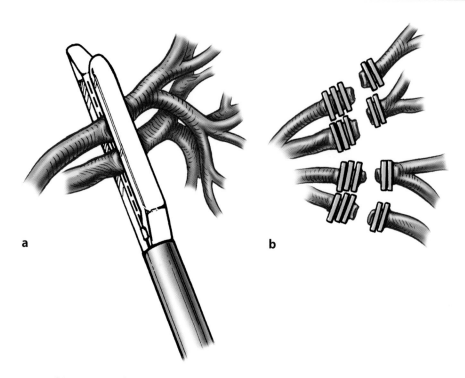

Fig. 12.12 (**b**) Division of the splenic vessels: (**a**) firing of the cutter and simultaneous control of both vessels; or (**b**) separate control of the artery and vein using large clips

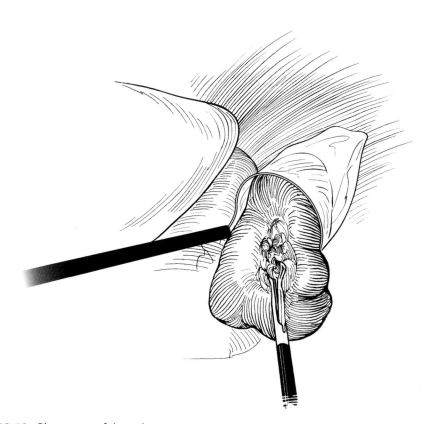

Fig. 12.13 Placement of the spleen into a retrieval bag

Final Steps of the Procedure

The ports are replaced. The area of the spleen is carefully checked for hemostasis. A drain is very rarely needed. This depends on the surgeon's experience and in particular on the degree of trauma to the tail of the pancreas during the dissection. If a drain is used, it should be taken out through a separate incision to avoid herniation of the small bowel while removing the drain through a large port site.

■ **Posterior Approach.** Laparoscopic splenectomy can also be performed via a posterior approach. The benefit of this approach is improved exposure of the hilar vessels compared to the anterior approach; however, in the anterior approach, the hilar vessels are controlled earlier in the procedure, which reduces the risk of uncontrollable bleeding later in the procedure.

The procedure follows these key steps:

- Division of the splenocolic ligament.
- Division of the inferior pole vessels.
- Division of the phrenic attachments.
- Exposure and division of the hilar vessels.
- Division of the short gastric vessels.
- Extraction of the spleen in a bag.

The surgeon begins the procedure by taking down the inferior pole vessels, as described for the anterior approach. After division of these vessels, the spleen is gently retracted medially and the splenophrenic ligament is divided using the harmonic shears (Fig. 12.14). This dissection continues superiorly until the short gastric vessels are encountered. Careful dissection of the splenorenal ligament is done at this point, with extreme attention given to avoid injury to the left adrenal gland. Next, the short gastric vessels are divided using the harmonic shears and clips as needed. The hilar vessels will now be in view, and can be dissected with a right angle dissector before being divided separately or together with a vascular endo cutter (Fig. 12.15). Next, the short gastric vessels are divided using the harmonic shears. The rest of the operation is performed as described in anterior approach.

■ **Post Operative Course.** The postoperative course following laparoscopic splenectomy is straightforward. Amylase and lipase levels should be checked on the first postoperative day to ensure there has been no pancreatic injury during the operation. A clear liquid diet is initiated if the levels are normal, and the patient can be discharged home once the diet has been tolerated.

■ **Management of Complications.** Bleeding constitutes a major problem. Two etiologies are possible:

- Bleeding from an unnamed vessel, such as a short gastric vessel or a branch of the inferior or superior pole vessels.
- Bleeding from a major vessel such as the splenic artery or vein.
- Bleeding from a splenic injury.

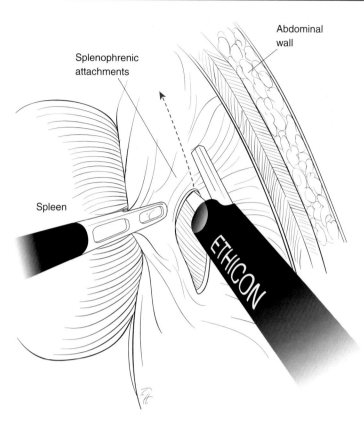

Fig. 12.14 Posterior approach for laparoscopic splenectomy; initial division of the spleno-phrenic ligament

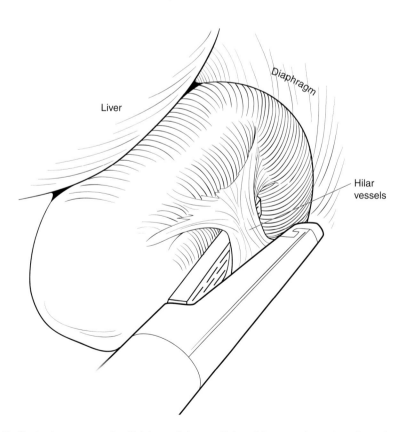

Fig. 12.15 Posterior approach; division of the pedicle with a stapler using the white vascular load

Control of an Unnamed Vessel

Control of an unnamed vessel should always be attempted and is usually successful. The first step is to pull back on the scope to protect the lens from blood. The vessel is then clamped using an atraumatic grasper. The grasper should be long and flat without teeth. Irrigation and aspiration of the surgical site should follow to evaluate the rate of bleeding. If the bleeding has been controlled, clips are placed appropriately. Sometimes, electrocautery will control the situation and allow safe placement of the clips. Compression using a laparoscopic 2 × 2 cm gauze can control the bleeding, allowing the operative site to be cleaned in preparation for hemostasis.

Control of a Major Vessel

The situation is different when a major vessel is injured. Examples are the splenic vein or artery, or the direct terminal branches of the main trunk. Flow is usually very high in these vessels, and blood reaching the left upper quadrant of the abdomen will obscure the view. In these circumstances, one can try to control the bleeding using the steps described previously, using a larger atraumatic instrument such as a bowel clamp to grasp the whole hilum. If this is not successful, it is usually wise to convert the patient rapidly through an open left subcostal incision.

Splenic Injury

Another possibility is an injury to the spleen itself during the dissection. A forceful retraction, for example, can tear the capsule. Although resultant bleeding may obscure the dissection, simple compression with a 2 × 2-cm surgical gauze together with appropriate electrocautery should control bleeding. If a combination of bleeding from the spleen and a minor vessel occurs, it is not possible to control both at the same time. It is recommended to either grab the bleeding vessel with a grasper while cauterizing the capsule, or control the capsular bleeding with a 2 × 2 gauze and compression while the bleeding vessel is clipped.

Maneuver of Last Resort During Bleeding of the Hilar Vessels

In the event of a splenic injury in traditional open surgery, the surgeon rapidly mobilizes the splenic attachments after inserting a large piece of gauze to compress the hilum. The surgeon's left hand retracts the splenic handle and the right hand clamps the vessels "en bloc" using large and long Kelly clamps. The same maneuvers can be realized laparoscopically if the surgeon and assistant have very good laparoscopic skills.

The hilum is compressed using a large 4 × 4 gauze and the bleeding controlled. As the short gastric vessels and the inferior attachments are already divided, the surgeon should promptly divide the phrenic attachments to mobilize the spleen. Once the spleen is mobilized, the assistant can retract the whole spleen superiorly with an open fan retractor, and the surgeon fires one or two shots of a linear cutter with vascular staples.

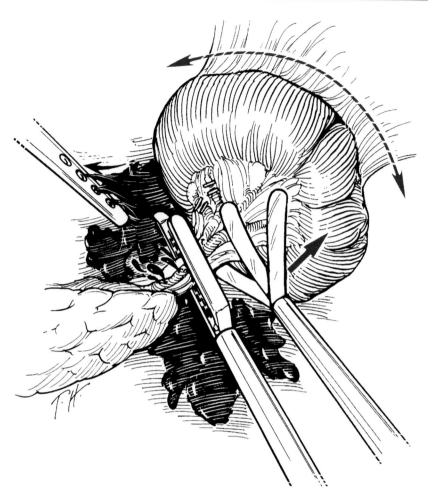

Fig. 12.16 Maneuver in the event of massive bleeding: Exposure of the hilum using a fan retractor with traction on the spleen to expose the spleno-pancreatic groove and the introduction of a stapler

This should be done quickly and staying as close as possible to the spleen to avoid pancreatic injury (Fig. 12.16).

If this maneuver is not successful, conversion to an open procedure should be initiated.

Partial Splenectomy

It is also possible to perform a partial laparoscopic splenectomy. In order to accomplish this, it is important to identify the inferior pole vessels, or any vessel per se, that is supplying the territory that has to be removed. Once the vessel is isolated using a right angle dissector, clips are placed and the vessel is divided, immediately producing a zone of ischemia in the spleen (Fig. 12.17). Once this has been achieved, harmonic shears are used to perform a partial splenectomy. Our preference is to use harmonic shears as they allow permanent hemostasis. It is important to leave 2 or 3 mm of zonal ischemia tissue on the remaining healthy spleen, and divide the spleen in the ischemic territory to avoid massive bleeding (Fig. 12.18). Once the partial splenectomy is performed, fibrin sealant is sprayed on the remaining tissue to further enhance homeostasis. The specimen will be removed as described previously.

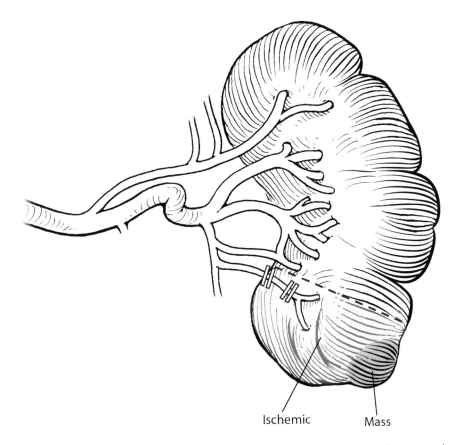

Ischemic   Mass

Fig. 12.17 Partial splenectomy. Ligation of the inferior polar vessels in this example that delineates a segmental zone of ischemia

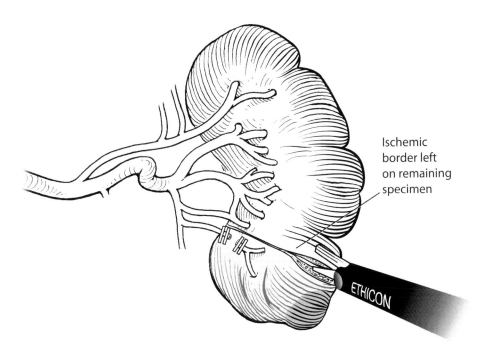

Ischemic border left on remaining specimen

Fig. 12.18 Partial splenectomy. Division of the splenic parenchyma using the harmonic shears, just beneath the line of ischemic demarcation

Hand Assisted Laparoscopic Splenectomy (HALS)

In the case of splenomegaly, as defined by a spleen over 20 cm in size, it is possible to use a hand-assisted technique (HALS). An incision is made for the nondominant hand the same size as the surgeon's glove size (7.5 → 7.5 cm, 8 → 8 cm, etc.), and a gelport is inserted to allow comfortable manipulation of the spleen (Fig. 12.19). It is important to place this incision rather away from the camera on the right side of the patient to avoid interaction between the hand and the scope. The procedure is then performed as described above.

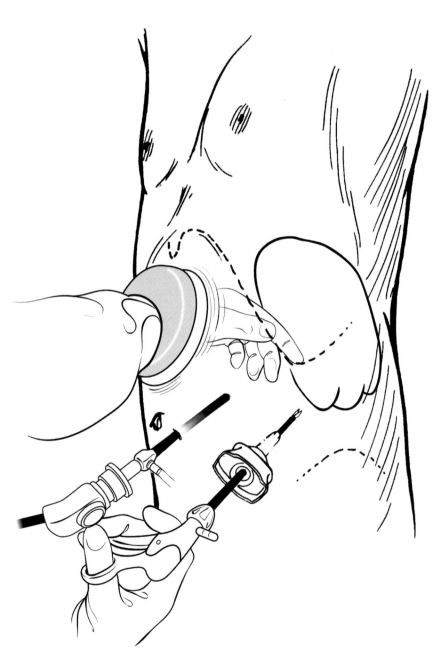

Fig. 12.19 Hand assisted laparoscopic surgery (HALS) for splenomegaly. The nondominant hand of the surgeon is introduced here

This procedure is illustrated in Fig. 12.20. The first step of the splenectomy is the mobilization of the inferior aspect of the spleen, dividing the phrenic attachments of the colon. The next step is the mobilization of the phrenic attachment of the spleen. The superior aspect of the spleen is then separated from the diaphragm. Once this is done, the short gastric vessels are taken down, exposing the pale tissue of the pancreatic tail. Alternatively, this mobilization of the spleen can be performed after the control of the splenic vessels and the division of the pancreatic tail. This has the advantage of keeping the spleen hanging on the diaphragm.

Distal Splenopancreatectomy

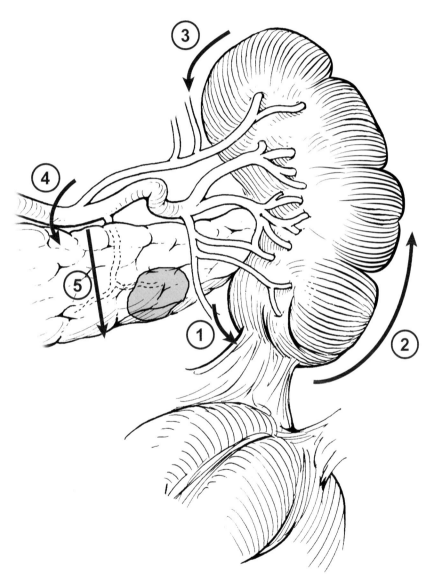

Fig. 12.20 Distal splenopancreatectomy steps: *1* mobilization of the inferior splenic pole; *2* division of the splenohepatic ligament; *3* mobilization of the superior pole of the spleen; *4* control of the splenic vessels at the superior aspect of the pancreatic tail; *5* division of the pancreatic tail. Alternatively, *1, 2, 3* can be performed after *4* and *5*

Slowly and carefully, the splenic artery and vein are identified. Sometimes it is possible to dissect both *en bloc*, but in most cases the splenic artery and the splenic vein are divided separately. Using the right angle dissector, the vessels are identified, dissected out, and divided using clips; it is indeed safer to place large clips than use a vascular linear stapler. The pancreatectomy is then completed using one firing of the linear cutter, 45 blue with seamguard (WL Gore Flagstaf, AZ) (Fig. 12.21). Hemeostasis is rechecked and any bleeding site is sutured to minimize the risk of pancreatic leak. The specimen is placed in a bag and removed.

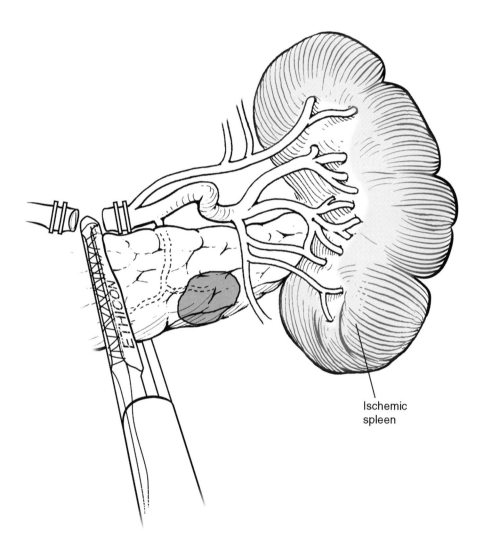

Ischemic spleen

Fig. 12.21 Stapling of the pancreatic tail using a stapler with a blue cartridge and reinforcement with Seamguard

Beanes S, Emil S, Kosi M, Applebaum H, Atkinson J (1995) A comparison of laparoscopic versus open splenectomy in children. Am Surg 61(10):908–910

Brunt LM, Langer JC, Quasebarth MA, Whitman ED (1996) Comparative analysis of laparo scopic versus open splenectomy. Am J Surg 172(5):596–599

Cadiere GB, Verroken R, Himpens J, Bruyns J, Efira M, De Wit S (1994) Operative strategy in laparoscopic splenectomy. J Am Coil Surg 179(6):668–672

Danno K, Ikeda M, Sekimoto M, Sugimoto T, Takemasa I, Yamamoto H, Doki Y, Monden M, Mori M (2009) Diameter of splenic vein is a risk factor for portal or splenic vein thrombosis after laparoscopic splenectomy. Surgery 145(5):457–464

Delaitre B (1995) Laparoscopic splenectomy: the 'hanged spleen' technique. Surg Endosc 9:528–529

Diaz J, Eisenstat M, Chung R (1997) A case-controlled study of laparoscopic splenectomy. Am J Surg 173(4):348–350

Duperier T, Brody F, Felsher J, Walsh RM, Rosen M, Ponsky J (2004) Predictive factors for successful laparoscopic splenectomy in patients with immune thrombocytopenic purpura. Arch Surg 139(1):61–66

Flowers JL, Lefor AT, Steers J, Heyman M, Graham SM, Imbembo AL (1996) Laparoscopic splenectomy in patients with hematologic diseases. Ann Surg 224(1):19–28

Glasgow RE, Yee LF, Mulvihill SJ (1997) Laparoscopic splenectomy. The emerging standard. Surg Endosc 11(2):108–112

Grahn SW, Alvarez J III, Kirkwood K (2006) Trends in laparoscopic splenectomy for massive splenomegaly. Arch Surg 141(8):755–756

Hashizume M, Sugimachi K, Kitano S et al (1994) Laparoscopic splenectomy. Am J Surg 167(6):611–614

Kaiser A, Umbach T, Katkhouda N (2002) Predictors of outcome after laparoscopic splenectomy. Probl Gen Surg 19:95–101

Katkhouda N, Hurwitz M (1999) Laparoscopic splenectomy for hematologic disease. Adv Surg 33:141–161

Katkhouda N, Hurwitz MB, Rivera RT, Chandra M, Waldrep DJ, Gugenheim J, Mouiel J (1998) Laparoscopic splenectomy: outcome and efficacy in 103 consecutive patients. Ann Surg 228(4):568–578

Katkhouda N, Le Goff D, Tricarico A, Castillo L (1988) Hydatid cyst of the pancreas responsible for chronic recurrent pancreatitis. La Presse Médicale 38:2021–2024 (in French)

Katkhouda N, Manhas S, Umbach TW, Kaiser A (2001) Laparoscopic splenectomy. J Laparoendosc Surg 11:383–390

Katkhouda N, Mavor E (2000) Laparoscopic splenectomy. Surg Clin North Am 80: 1285–1297

Katkhouda N, Mouiel J (1986) Pancreatic cancer in mother and daughter. Lancet 8509(9):74

Katkhouda N, Tricarico A, Mouiel J (1988) Acute pancreatitis: the role of biliary millilithiasis. Urgentis Chirurgiae Commentaria 11:27–31 (in Italian)

Katkhouda N, Umbach T, Kaiser A (2002) Splenectomy: anterior laparoscopic approach. Probl Gen Surg 19:24–28

Katkhouda N, Waldrep D, Feinstein D, Soliman H, Stain S, Ortega A, Mouiel J (1996) Unresolved issues in laparoscopic splenectomy. Am J Surg 172:585–590

Liang MK, Marks JL (2007) Postsplenectomy portal, mesenteric, and splenic vein thrombosis. Arch Surg 142(6):575

Miles WF, Greig JD, Wilson RG, Nixon SJ (1996) Technique of laparoscopic splenectomy with a powered vascular linear stapler. Br J Surg 83(9):1212–1214

Mouiel J, Katkhouda N (1992) Endo-laparoscopic treatment of pancreatic cancer. Surg Laparosc Endosc 2:241–243

Phillips EH, Carroll BJ, Fallas MJ (1994) Laparoscopic splenectomy. Surg Endosc 8(8):931–933

Poulin EC, Thibault C (1995) Laparoscopic splenectomy for massive splenomegaly: operative technique and case report. Can J Surg 38(1):69–72

Poulin BC, Thibault C, Mamazza J (1995) Laparoscopic splenectomy. Surg Endosc 9(2):172–176

Rege RV, Merriam LT, Joehi RJ (1996) Laparoscopic splenectomy. Surg Clin N Am 76(3): 459–468

Rhodes M, Rudd M, O'Rourke N, Nathanson L, Fielding G (1995) Laparoscopic splenectomy and lymph node biopsy for hematologic disorders. Ann Surg 222(1):43–46

Rothenberg SS (1996) Laparoscopic splenectomy using the harmonic scalpel. J Laparoendosc Surg 6(suppl 1):S61–S63.

Rudowski WJ (1995) Laparoscopic splenectomy. Am J Surg 169(2):282–283

Saldinger PF, Matthews JB, Mowschenson PM, Hodin RA (1996) Stapled laparoscopic sple nectomy: initial experience. J Am Coil Surg 182(5):459–461

Sampath S, Meneghetti AT, MacFarlane JK, Nguyen NH, Benny WB, Panton ON (2007) An 18-year review of open and laparoscopic splenectomy for idiopathic thrombocytopenic purpura. Am J Surg 193(5):580–583

Schlinkert RT, Mann D (1995) Laparoscopic splenectomy offers advantages in selected patients with immune thrombocytopenic purpura. Am J Surg 170(6):624–626

Smith CD, Meyer TA, Goretsky MJ (1996) Laparoscopic splenectomy by the lateral approach: a safe and effective alternative to open splenectomy for hematologic diseases. Surgery 120(5):789–794

Trias M, Targarona EM, Balague C (1996) Laparoscopic splenectomy: an evolving technique. A comparison between anterior and lateral approaches. Surg Endosc 10(4):389–392

Uranus S, Pfeifer J, Schauer C et al (1995) Laparoscopic partial splenic resection. Surg Laparosc Endosc 5(2):133–136

Watson DI, Coventry BJ, Chin T, Gill PG, Malycha P (1997) Laparoscopic versus open splenectomy for immune thrombocytopenic purpura. Surgery 121(1):18–22

Yee LF, Carvajal SH, de Lorimier AA, Mulvihill ST (1995) Laparoscopic splenectomy. The initial experience at University of California, San Francisco. Arch Surg 130(8):874–877Incisional

Adrenalectomy 13

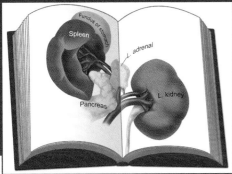

Principles

Laparoscopic adrenalectomy, whether performed via the transabdominal approach or the totally retroperitoneal technique, has two main principles:

- Extracapsular dissection of the gland to avoid rupture of the adrenal and seeding of tumor cells in the retroperitoneum.
- A meticulous dissection technique to achieve perfect hemostasis, with particular attention to ligation of the adrenal vein.

Left Adrenalectomy

The patient is lifted on a bean-bag with safe padding to avoid compression injury. The patient is placed in full right lateral decubitus for a left adrenalectomy (Fig. 13.1) and 60° right side up for a right adrenalectomy (Fig. 13.2). The operating table is flexed as much as possible to increase the distance between the costal margin and the iliac crest. The patient who is undergoing a left adrenalectomy with a prominent iliac crest may also be positioned at 60°, left side up so that the iliac crest does not obstruct movement of the camera and instruments. The operating table must be capable of manipulation in all directions, especially reverse Trendelenburg.

The operation begins with insertion of a Veress needle into the abdominal cavity through the umbilicus, and after a confirmatory test, the pressure is regulated at 15 mmHg. A 30° laparoscope is inserted to explore the abdomen and check for adhesions that would necessitate an enterolysis.

N. Katkhouda, *Advanced Laparoscopic Surgery*,
DOI: 10.1007/978-3-540-74843-4_13, © Springer-Verlag Berlin Heidelberg 2011

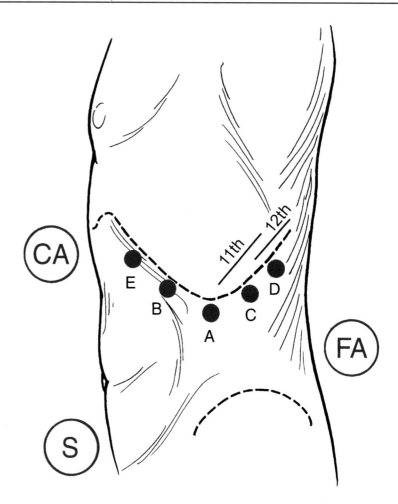

Fig. 13.1 Port positions for left adrenalectomy: *A* 30-degree scope; *B* surgeon's left hand; *C* surgeon's right hand; *D* grasper of first assistant; *E* irrigation or fan retractor. *S* surgeon; *FA* first assistant; *CA* camera assistant

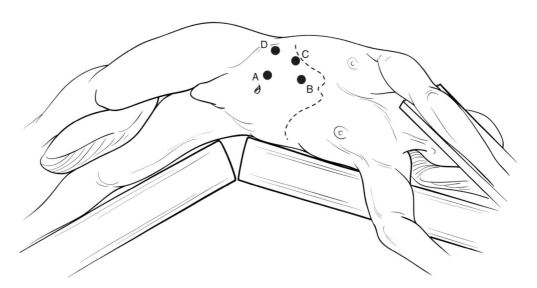

Fig. 13.2 Port placement for right adrenalectomy. *A* camera; *B* right hand of surgeon; *C* left hand of surgeon; *d* grasper for assistant

To begin, four trocars are inserted in a triangulated fashion (Fig. 13.1). The first is a port for the camera in front of the 11th rib, the second is placed at the midclavicular line for the surgeon's left hand, the third is positioned at the anterior axillary line for the surgeon's right hand, and the fourth port is located at the posterior axillary line. Occasionally, a fifth subxiphoid trocar may be required for suctioning or retraction of the spleen.

The left adrenalectomy can be compared to opening a book, where the left adrenal gland is located on the spine of the book, and the spleen and left kidney are the covers of the book. The analogy is to open the book and access its spine (by incising the splenic attachments and allowing the spleen to drop medially) (Fig. 13.3). The splenic flexure of the colon is mobilized by incising its lateral peritoneal attachments from the inferior part of the spleen using a harmonic scalpel. The splenophrenic ligament is then divided 1 cm lateral to the spleen by a very gentle medial retraction of the spleen, followed by generous division of the splenophrenic ligament (Fig. 13.4). This is the *key to laparoscopic left adrenalectomy*, as it allows the spleen to fall medially and exposes the left kidney. Placing the patient in steep reverse Trendelenburg improves the exposure by causing inferior displacement of the intestine and any fluid that accumulated during the operation.

Dissection then proceeds superiorly between the spleen and the kidney towards the diaphragm until the fundus of stomach is visualized, at which point the adrenal gland should come into view between the spleen and the left kidney (Fig. 13.3). The adrenal gland itself is distinguishable from surrounding retroperitoneal fat by its golden color and granular texture on the cortical surface, in contrast to the brown smooth surface of the kidney.

The superior pole of the adrenal gland is mobilized first (Fig. 13.5). The medial aspect of the gland where most of the adrenal blood supply enters is then mobilized. Mobilization of the adrenal gland and control of its blood supply are accomplished using

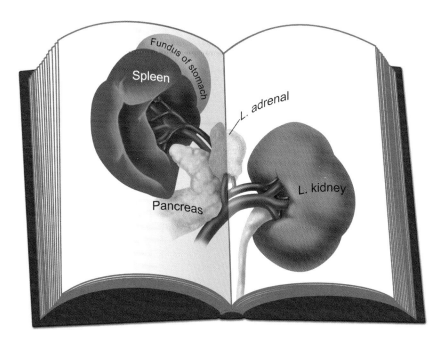

Fig. 13.3 Left adrenal gland located on the spine of the book

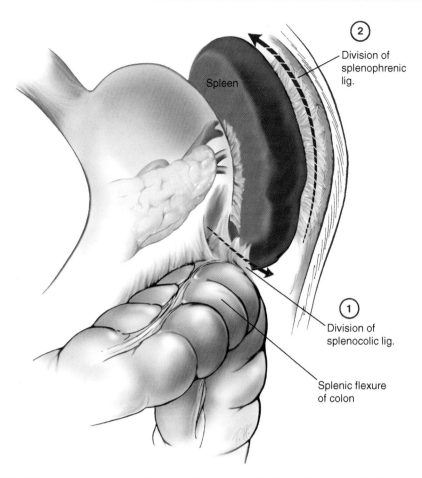

Fig. 13.4 Dissection route for left adrenalectomy: *1* division of splenocolic ligament; *2* division of splenophrenic ligament

a harmonic scalpel. Clips are placed for larger arterial branches as needed. Special attention is warranted to avoid entering the adrenal parenchyma, which will result in bleeding and possible seeding of tumor cells. Parenchymal bleeding can be controlled using the spatula connected to electocautery.

A second atraumatic grasper should be used to manipulate the adrenal gland. Gently, traction is provided by either depressing the kidney or by retracting the adrenal itself, taking care not to disrupt the capsule of the gland. The laparoscope and all other dissecting instruments should be moved as necessary between the ports to maximize visualization and provide ideal angles for efficient dissection.

As the dissection progresses inferiorly, the central adrenal vein will come into view (Fig. 13.5). The left adrenal vein is several centimeters long, and after exiting the gland anteriorly, it courses obliquely to empty into the left renal vein. The inferior phrenic vein usually joins the left adrenal vein within 15 mm of its entry into the renal vein. Surgical control of the left adrenal vein is the most important and delicate part of the procedure; its course differs from the right adrenal vein, which is shorter (5–10 mm long) and exits the gland medially to enter the posterior medial aspect of the inferior vena cava (Fig. 13.6). Sometimes, a second adrenal vein is seen on the right entering either the IVC or a hepatic vein. The adrenal vein is then double-clipped and divided, and the lateral aspect of the vein

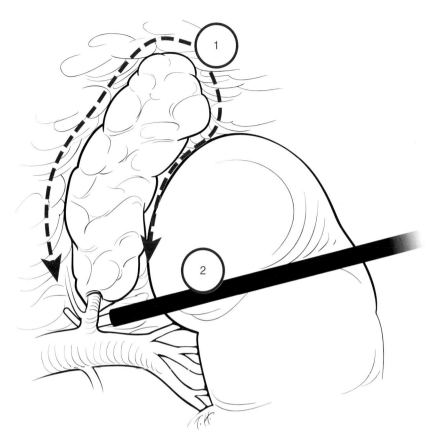

Fig. 13.5 Dissection of the superior aspect of the left adrenal gland *1* and mobilization of the gland itself. Control of the left adrenal vein performed next *2*

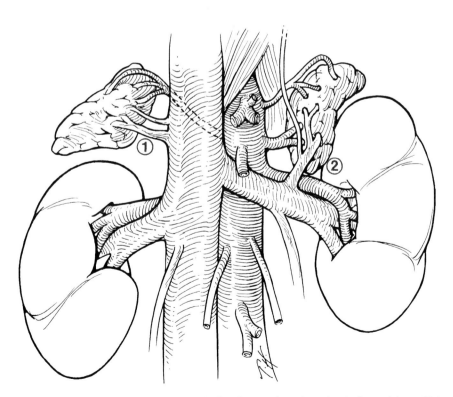

Fig. 13.6 Surgical anatomy of the adrenal glands: *1* right adrenal vein branching off the IVC; *2* left adrenal vein branching off the left renal vein

can now be mobilized. Next, the inferior aspect of the gland is mobilized from the superior pole of the kidney, and the gland is placed in a special retrieval bag. The retroperitoneal operative bed is finally irrigated and inspected for bleeding using a 2 × 2 gauze. Tisseel can be sprayed to improve hemostasis. The spleen is replaced into its original location. Trocar sites should be closed if dilatation of a port site was necessary to remove the specimen.

Right Adrenalectomy

The procedure is similar to that of left adrenalectomy except that modification is required to take into account the anatomic differences. This operation is more difficult due to the position of the right adrenal gland behind the liver, the proximity of the inferior vena cava, and the anatomy of the adrenal vein. Manipulation of the adrenal vein is especially hazardous on the right side, where laceration of the vein can lead to tearing of the inferior vena cava and potentially catastrophic hemorrhage.

Following insufflation of the abdomen, the camera port is placed above the umbilicus and to the right approximately 10 cm below the costal margin. The best view is when

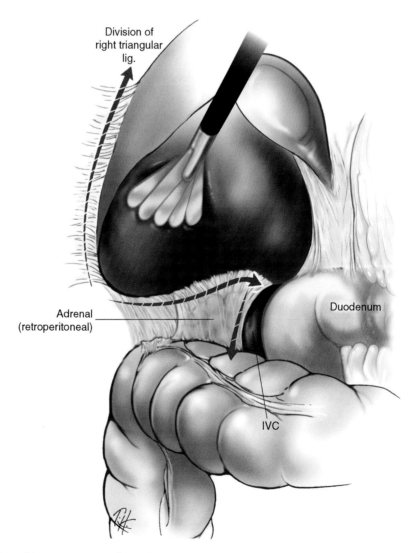

Fig. 13.7 Dissection route for right adrenalectomy: (**a**) division of adhesions between the hepatic flexure of the colon and the liver; (**b**) division of right triangular ligament of the liver

the gallbladder is in the upper right side of the screen, the duodenum in the lower right, the liver superiorly and the kidney on the left. Two additional trocars are placed in a triangulated fashion on each side of the camera close to the costal margin. The forth trocar is placed right under the costal margin for retraction of the liver, and another trocar can be placed in left flank for assistance (Fig. 13.2).

For right laparoscopic adrenalectomy, *the right triangular ligament of the liver is the key to safe dissection,* and must be incised generously to allow retraction of the right lobe of the liver with a fan retractor (Fig. 13.7). The continuous superior retraction of the liver is very important for exposure of the right adrenal gland. The right triangular ligament is carefully divided using the harmonic scalpel. This dissection continues superiorly until the anterior surface of the right adrenal is visualized. One should be careful with the small hepatic veins that enter the vena cava at this point. The hepatic flexure of the colon is mobilized and the colon can be pushed down to allow entry into the retroperitoneal space if additional exposure is needed. The duodenum is mobilized to expose the inferior vena cava as necessary. This is done using a small 2×2 cm gauze and careful blunt dissection. A peanut dissector is also useful here.

The superior and medial poles of the adrenal gland are mobilized first (Fig. 13.8). As the dissection proceeds along the lateral aspect of the IVC, the right adrenal vein is

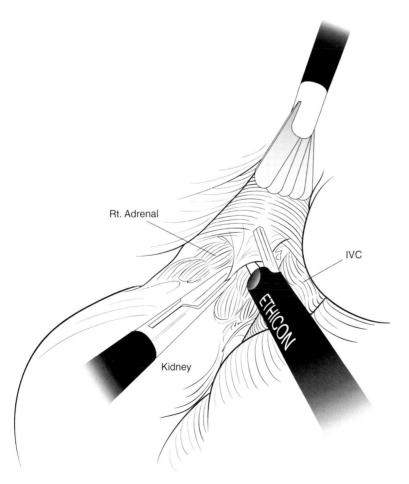

Fig. 13.8 Mobilization of the superior and medial paracaval aspect of the right adrenal gland

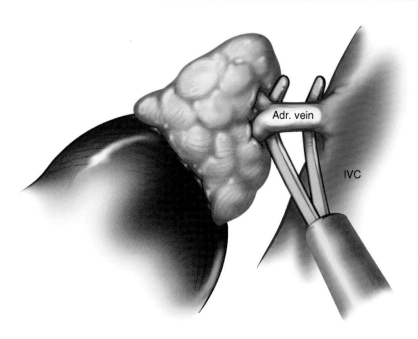

Fig. 13.9 Exposure of the right middle adrenal vein using a right angle dissector

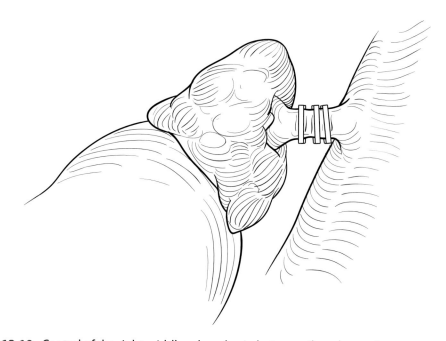

Fig. 13.10 Control of the right middle adrenal vein between three large clips

encountered as it enters the posterior medial aspect of IVC. At all times, care should be taken not to cauterize the adrenal vein; instead, the vein is dissected using right-angled dissectors (Fig. 13.9). In contrast to the left side, on the right side the adrenal vein is *short* and exits the gland medially to enter the posterior medial aspect of the inferior vena cava (Fig. 13.6). Occasionally, a second adrenal vein is seen on the right, entering either the inferior vena cava or a hepatic vein. The complex anatomy of this area is the biggest hazard of this operation, and confusion here may result in massive hemorrhage.

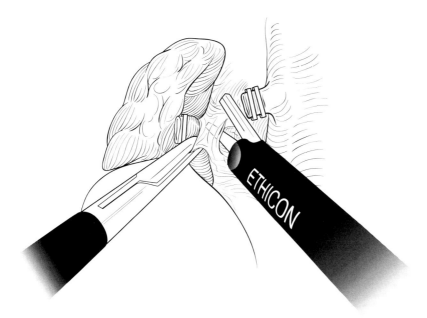

Fig. 13.11 After ligation of the adrenal vein, mobilization of the gland from the medial to the lateral aspect

The adrenal vein is controlled and divided between large clips (Fig. 13.10). An intracorporeal tie can be placed carefully if clips are not satisfactory.

When the adrenal vein has been divided, the adrenal gland is freed of its remaining attachments inferiorly and posteriorly, from the medial to its most lateral aspect (Fig. 13.11), and the operation is completed as described for left adrenalectomy. Tisseel spray can be used for better hemostasis of exposed retroperitoneum.

Potential hazards include injury to the IVC or a clip falling off the adrenal vein stump. An atraumatic flat clamp can be used to control the bleeding, and larger vascular clamps designed for laparoscopic vascular surgery may be used if available. Otherwise, swift conversion to open surgery and hemostasis is required.

Selected Further Reading

Berber E, Tellioglu G, Harvey A, Mitchell J, Milas M, Siperstein A (2009) Comparison of laparoscopic transabdominal lateral versus posterior retroperitoneal adrenalectomy. Surgery 146(4):621–625

Brunt LM, Doherty GM, Norton TA, Soper NJ, Quasebarth MA, Moley JF (1996) Laparoscopic adrenalectomy compared to open adrenalectomy for benign adrenal neoplasms. J Am Coil Surg 183(1):1–10

Deans GT, Kappadia R, Wedgewood K, Royston CM, Brough WA (1995) Laparoscopic adrenalectomy. Br J Surg 82(7):994–995

Duh QY, Siperstein AE, Clark OH et al (1996) Comparison of the lateral and posterior approaches. Laparoscopic adrenalectomy. Arch Surg 131(8):870–875

Fahey TJ III, Reeve TS, Deibridge L (1994) Adrenalectomy: expanded indications for the extraperitoneal approach. Aust NZ J Surg 64(7):494–497

Fernandez-Cruz L (1996) Laparoscopic adrenal surgery. Br J Surg 83(6):721–723

Fletcher DR, Beiles CB, Hardy KS (1994) Laparoscopic adrenalectomy. Aust NZ J Surg 64(6):427–430

Gagner M, Lacroix A, Bolte E, Pomp A (1994) Laparoscopic adrenalectomy. The importance of a flank approach in the lateral decubitus position. Surg Endosc 8(2):135–138

Guazzoni G, Montorsi F, Bocciardi A et al (1995) Transperitoneal laparoscopic versus open adrenalectomy for benign hyperfunctioning adrenal tumors: a comparative study. J Urol 153(5):1597–1600

Henneman D, Chang Y, Hodin RA, Berger DL (2009) Effect of laparoscopy on the indications for adrenalectomy. Arch Surg 144(3):255–259

Jacobs JK, Goldstein RE, Geer RJ (1997) Laparoscopic adrenalectomy: a new standard of care. Ann Surg 225(5):495–502

Kalan MM, Tillou G, Kulick A, Wilcox CS, Garcia AI (2004) Performing laparoscopic adrenalectomy safely. Arch Surg 139(11):1243–1247

Kim AW, Quiros RM, Maxhimer JB, El-Ganzouri AR, Prinz RA (2004) Outcome of laparoscopic adrenalectomy for pheochromocytomas vs aldosteronomas. Arch Surg 139(5):526–529

Lee JA, Zarnegar R, Shen WT, Kebebew E, Clark OH, Duh QY (2007) Adrenal incidentaloma, borderline elevations of urine or plasma metanephrine levels, and the "subclinical" pheochromocytoma. Arch Surg 142(9):870–873

Lombardi CP, Raffaelli M, De Crea C, Sollazzi L, Perilli V, Cazzato MT, Bellantone R (2008) Endoscopic adrenalectomy: Is there an optimal operative approach? Results of a single-center case-control study. Surgery 144(6):1008–1014

MacGillivray DC, Shichman SJ, Ferrer FA, Maichoff CD (1996) A comparison of open vs laparoscopic adrenalectomy. Surg Endosc 10(10):987–990

Nash PA, Leibovitch I, Donohue JP (1995) Adrenalectomy via the dorsal approach: a bench mark for laparoscopic adrenalectomy. J Urol 154(5):1652–1654

Perrier ND, Kennamer DL, Bao R, Jimenez C, Grubbs EG, Lee JE, Evans DB (2008) Posterior retroperitoneoscopic adrenalectomy: preferred technique for removal of benign tumors and isolated metastases. Ann Surg 248(4):666–674

Pertsemlidis D (1995) Minimal-access versus open adrenalectomy. Surg Endosc 9(4):384–386

Prager G, Heinz-Peer G, Passler C, Kaczirek K, Scheuba C, Niederle B (2004) Applicability of laparoscopic adrenalectomy in a prospective study in 150 consecutive patients. Arch Surg 139(1):46–49

Schlinkert RT, van Heerden TA, Grant CS, Thompson GB, Segura JW (1995) Laparoscopic left adrenalectomy for aldosteronoma: early Mayo Clinic experience. Mayo Clin Proc 70(9):844–846

Skarsgard ED, Albanese CT (2005) The safety and efficacy of laparoscopic adrenalectomy in children. Arch Surg 140(9):905–908

Stuart RC, Chung SC, Lau JY et al (1995) Laparoscopic adrenalectomy. Br J Surg 82(11): 1498–1499

Toniato A, Boschin IM, Opocher G, Guolo A, Pelizzo M, Mantero F (2007) Is the laparoscopic adrenalectomy for pheochromocytoma the best treatment? Surgery 141(6): 723–727

Toniato A, Merante-Boschin I, Opocher G, Pelizzo MR, Schiavi F, Ballotta E (2009) Surgical versus conservative management for subclinical Cushing syndrome in adrenal incidentalomas: a prospective randomized study. Ann Surg 249(3):388–391

Bariatric Surgery 14

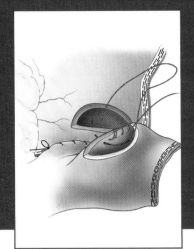

It is critical to differentiate patients based on shape in addition to BMI, and we have found that body habitus is more predictive of operative difficulty than BMI. For example, male diabetic patients with an apple shape are much more difficult operative cases than female patients with a high BMI but a pear shape body habitus. In this regard, we have identified a special trocar placement technique that takes this concept into consideration. The distance between the xyphoid process and the umbilicus before insufflation of the abdomen is called the XU distance. If the XU distance is less than 25 cm, it is possible to perform the operation with one regular set of trocars as depicted in Fig. 14.1. If the distance is greater than 25 cm, we recommend using the *advanced trocar placement*. This technique uses two sets of trocars, with the first set of triangulated trocars focused on the creation of jejunojejunostomy, and the second set placed cephalad to the first to perform the gastric part of the operation, as depicted in Fig. 14.2.

Another indicator of difficulty is a tense abdomen on physical examination. These patients need to lose 5% of their weight preoperatively to decrease the amount of intra-abdominal fat. There are four areas affected by weight loss: the omentum, the falciform ligament, the perigastric fat and last and most importantly, the liver. A fatty liver in a patient who has not lost weight will cover the stomach and make it very difficult to access the angle of His and staple the stomach safely (Fig. 14.3).

In some patients, there is a fold of skin right at the level of the umbilicus. Above this fold, there is often a protuberant and very thick abdominal wall. One should avoid placing trocars on or inferior to this fold, as it makes the operation more difficult. Instead, it is recommended to place the trocars above the fold.

Laparoscopic Roux-en-Y Gastric Bypass

N. Katkhouda, *Advanced Laparoscopic Surgery*,
DOI: 10.1007/978-3-540-74843-4_14, © Springer-Verlag Berlin Heidelberg 2011

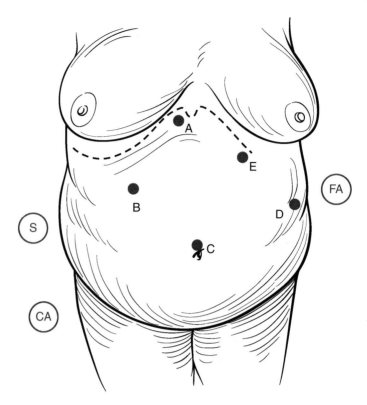

Fig. 14.1 Basic trocar placement for Roux-en-Y gastric bypass. *C* camera; *B* left hand of surgeon; *E* right hand of surgeon; *D* trocar for assistant; *A* liver retractor. *S* surgeon; *CA* camera assistant; *FA* first assistant

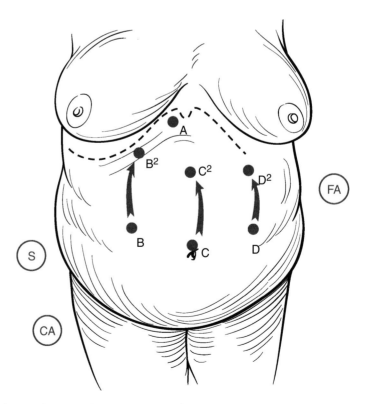

Fig. 14.2 Advanced trocar placement for Roux-en-Y gastric bypass. *B, C, D* moved to *B2, C2, D2* (*B* and *B2*, left hand of surgeon; *C* and *C2*, camera port; *D* and *D2*, right hand of surgeon)

A. - Obese patient

B - After significant weight loss

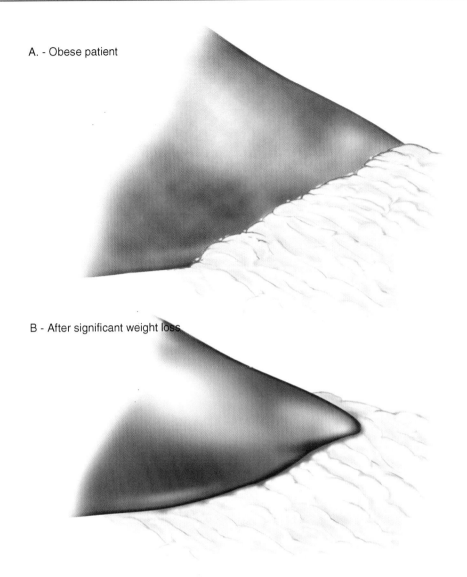

Fig. 14.3 Effect of preoperative weight loss on the fatty liver. A = before preoperative weight loss, the liver is swollen. B = after significant preoperative weight loss, the fatty liver "shrinks"

Patient Positioning

The patient is placed in the supine position with both arms out. Care must be taken not to extend the arms excessively to prevent brachial plexus injury. The beds should be specialized for bariatric patients with a footboard to avoid sliding during the procedure, especially in steep reverse Trendelenberg. Padding is very important secondary to the increased weight of the patient on pressure points. A Foley catheter is placed and an orogastric tube is inserted by the anesthesiologist, which will be removed prior to stapling the stomach.

Technique

The surgeon stands on the right of the patient, the camera assistant stands behind him, and the first assistant is on the opposite (left) side of the patient. The first step is insufflation of the abdomen. We believe that the easiest technique is the use of the Veress needle. This has been done safely in our experience of more than 1,000 cases. An optiview trocar is then inserted slightly above the umbilicus. Once the optiview trocar is in place, the right and left hand of the surgeon's ports are placed in a double triangulated fashion, as described in Chap. 1. The next trocar placed is used for retraction of the transverse colon. This same trocar will be used by the right hand of the surgeon during the gastric part of the operation. In case of difficulties, two 5-mm trocars are inserted for the assistant on the left side.

The next step is division of the greater omentum, which is performed using the harmonic shears. This reduces the distance the alimentary loop must travel to reach the stomach (Fig. 14.4). In the case of severe adhesions, we remove them by directing specific

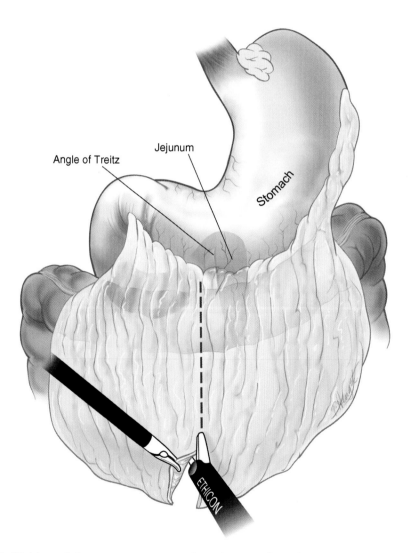

Fig. 14.4 Division of the greater omentum in order to reduce the hump for the positioning of the antecolic Roux-en-Y intestinal loop

trocars towards this task; the greater omentum can also be divided from right to left at the limit of the transverse colon, thereby sufficiently mobilizing the greater omentum to access the ligament of Treitz. Once the greater omentum is divided, clips are placed at the division to mark the site where the jejunal loop will be placed on the colon. The transverse colon is retracted using a Babcock grasper. The area of division of small bowel is identified approximately 20–25 cm from the angle of Treitz. The small bowel is exposed with the left hand using an atraumatic grasper; an assistant can help with counter-traction An Ethicon GIA-45 (white) is fired to transect the small bowel (Fig. 14.5). One and half firings of the GIA-45 white should divide the mesentery (Fig. 14.6). To avoid injuring

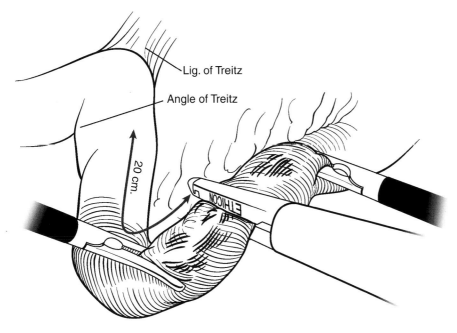

Fig. 14.5 Division of the jejunum 20–25 cm from the angle of Treitz using a white load

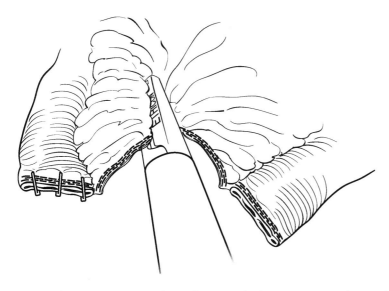

Fig. 14.6 Division of the mesentery with 1.5 firings with the 45 mm vascular stapler

the superior mesenteric artery, one should never fire more than two loads of the GIA-45 in the mesentery (Fig. 14.7). The next step is coagulation of any bleeding along the cut edges of the mesentery. It is extremely important to use electrocautery or clips to avoid postoperative bleeding. The harmonic shears are used to open up the crotch of this division to further extend the length of the alimentary loop. Occasionally, the proximal part of the Roux limb becomes ischemic due to stapling of the feeding vessels. Using another GIA-45 white, this piece of small bowel – like a Ravioli – will be transected where a pulsating artery is seen at the mesenteric border of the small bowel (Fig. 14.8). The proximal part of the cut intestine is marked using several clips placed along the staple line to avoid confusion when pulling the roux limb up. This provides orientation of the 100–150 cm loop. If the BMI is less than 50, a 100-cm loop is used, while a 150 cm loop is constructed if the BMI is greater than 50. A clip is placed distally, and the smallest possible opening is made using the harmonic shears (Fig. 14.9). The same opening is then created on the proximal part of the small bowel. At this point, the GIA-45 white is inserted, and the jejunojejunostomy is created. Stabilization of the stapler is performed using the stapler nearly closed to avoid widening the opening (Fig. 14.10). The jejunostomy is then closed. One Kaiser stitch – named after one of our attendings – is placed at the lower part of the enterotomy (Fig. 14.11), and the enterotomy is closed with a running 3–0 Prolene on an SH1, the best possible small needle (Fig. 14.12). The Kaiser stitch is tied to the running suture. The mesenteric window is closed using a running 3–0 nonabsorbable suture, minimizing the risk of internal hernias (Fig. 14.13). The area is thoroughly checked for bleeding. At this point, attention is directed to the second part of the operation (construction of the gastric pouch) (Fig. 14.14). The patient is placed in reverse Trendelenburg

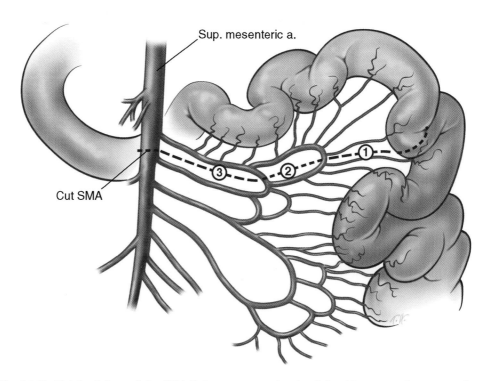

Fig. 14.7 Risk for injury of the SMA if three or more loads of the 45 mm stapler are used

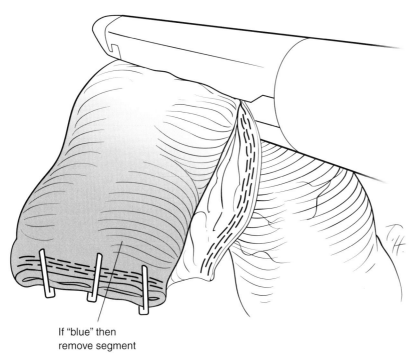

If "blue" then
remove segment

Fig. 14.8 Resection of an ischemic small bowel tip (resection of a "Ravioli")

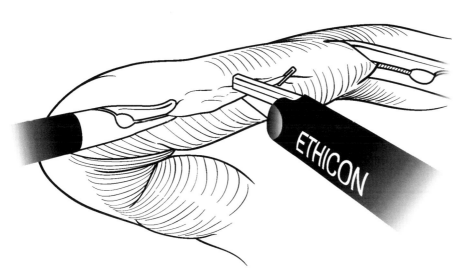

Fig. 14.9 Enterotomy for the jejunojejunostomy using the harmonic shears; the distal jejunum is marked with a clip

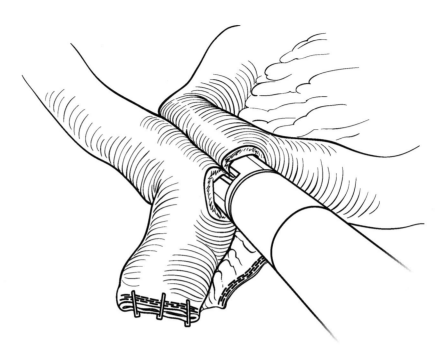

Fig. 14.10 Side to side jejunojejunostomy using the 45 mm vascular stapler. The proximal tip of the jejunum was marked with clips

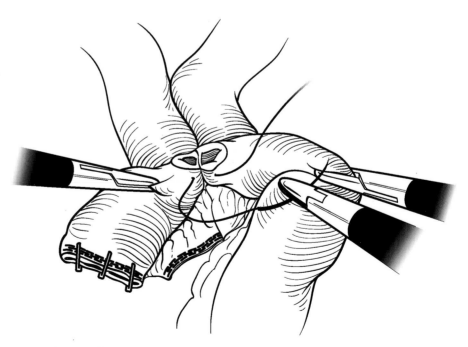

Fig. 14.11 Closure of the enterotomies using a running 3–0 Prolene on an SH1 needle. The proximal corener is closed using one interrupted stitch (the "Kaiser" stitch)

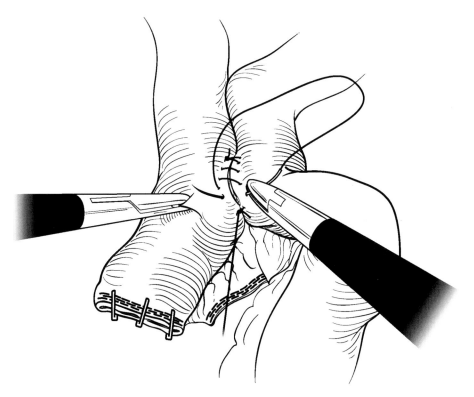

Fig. 14.12 Closure of the enterotomies using an extramucosal running 3–0 Prolene stitch

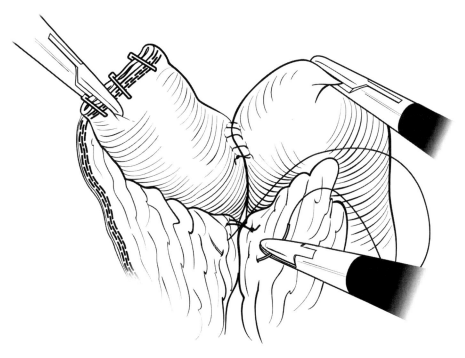

Fig. 14.13 Closure of the mesenteric defect using a running 2–0 Ethibond suture

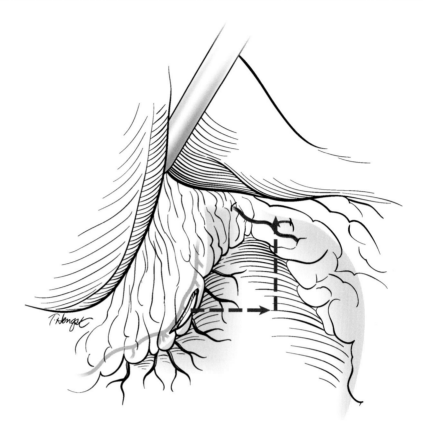

Fig. 14.14 Figure depicting the future gastric pouch

position. The liver is retracted superiorly after inserting the subxiphoid trocar. Mandatory preoperative weight loss will reduce the volume of a fatty liver, which enhances and eases the use of sophisticated instruments in all cases. The angle of His is identified to the left side of the fat pad and opened gently with the harmonic shears. The "L" retractor is then used to further open the angle of His. Next, the lesser curvature is identified slightly under the second gastric vein. The harmonic shears are used to open the lesser omentum close to the gastric wall. With the assistance of two graspers, the lesser sac is opened promptly without further dissection with the harmonic shears to minimize the risk of burn injury to the gastric wall (Fig. 14.15). At this point, with the right hand of the surgeon holding the L retractor inside the opening, a GIA-45 blue is fed through the window (Fig. 14.16). Before firing the stapler, the NG-tube is removed by the anesthesiologist, and then several firings of the GIA-45 blue will finish the creation of the gastric pouch vertically, and clips are placed along the staple line for hemostasis as needed. It is very important to *avoid a fold* during the first vertical firing at the intersection between the horizontal and vertical staple lines; such a fold can create a weak point, and is frequently the site of staple line disruption, especially when stapling the thick stomach of a male patient. This disruption can cause a postoperative leak (Fig. 14.17). The L-shaped retractor will always precede the introduction of the stapler (Fig. 14.18).

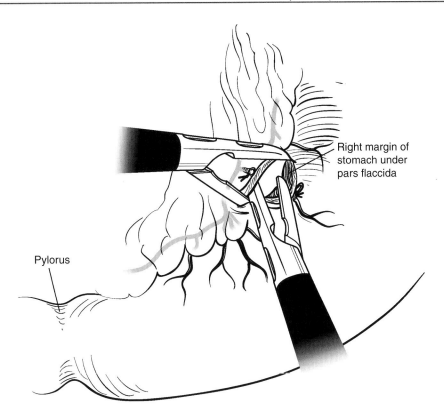

Fig. 14.15 Preparation of the firing of the first transverse cut; opening the retrogastric window medial to the nerve of Latarjet, using a maneuver with two atraumatic grasper forceps

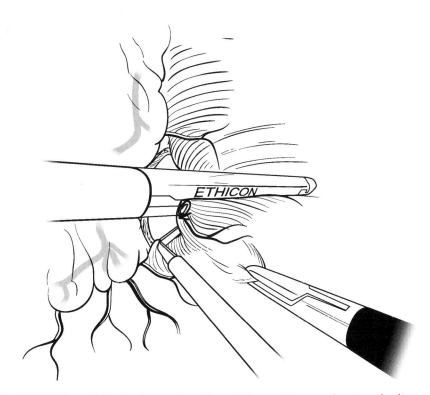

Fig. 14.16 Division of the horitzontal portion of the gastric pouch using the linear 45 mm stapler with blue loads. Note the inferior retraction of the grasper forceps of the assistant, and the placement of the right-angled "L" shaped retractor holding the gastric pouch, held by the right hand of the surgeon

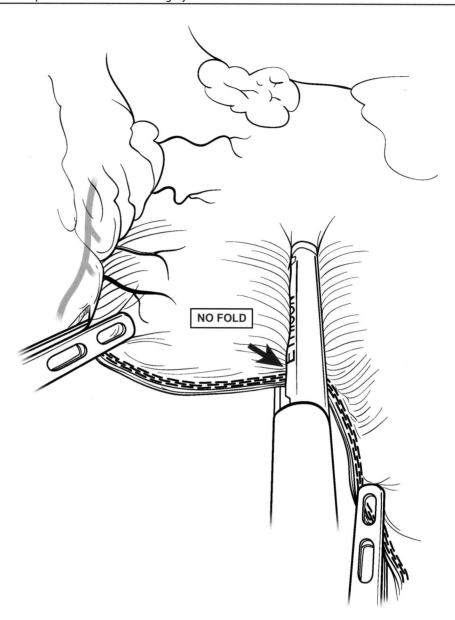

Fig. 14.17 Division of the vertical portion of the pouch; the 45 mm stapler is placed as *not* to create a fold at the intersection of the two staple lines

Occasionally, after the firing of the last load of staples (Fig. 14.19), there is a connection remaining between the pouch and the gastric remnant (Fig. 14.20). Cutting this tissue can result in a leak from this corner, and convert the angle of His to the angle of sorrow. Although it seems like a waste of a staple load, this tissue should also be divided with a stapler to make sure that there is no opening at the corner. Sometimes, after complete division of the stomach, there is a sharp angle at the corner of the pouch that can look dusky. This should be trimmed with another firing of the stapler. In female patients, we also use the Seamguard (Gore Inc, Flagstaff, AZ) to reinforce the staple lines and ensure hemostasis; however, we do not use the Seamguard with the first and last staple loads (technically at the corners), so that if there is a problem that needs to be fixed with a suture, the Seamguard is not in the way. In men, we often avoid using Seamguards due

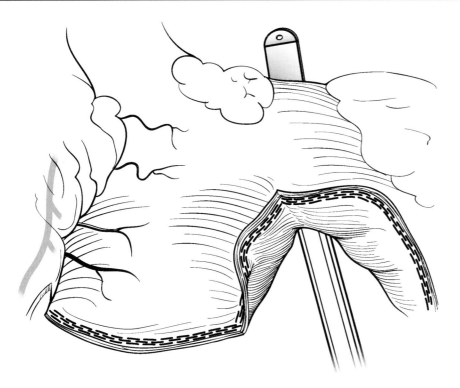

Fig. 14.18 Introduction of the "L" shaped retractor that emerges just lateral to the angle of His, the fat pad always left medially

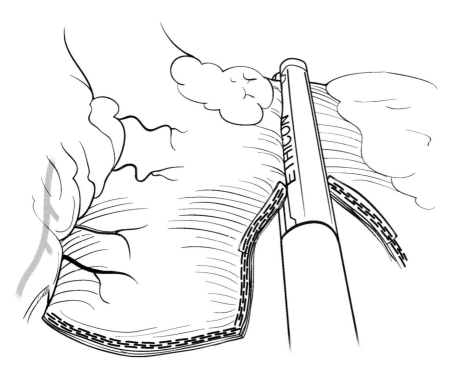

Fig. 14.19 Firing the stapler using Seamguard vicryl reinforcement; the tip of the stapler should always be visible

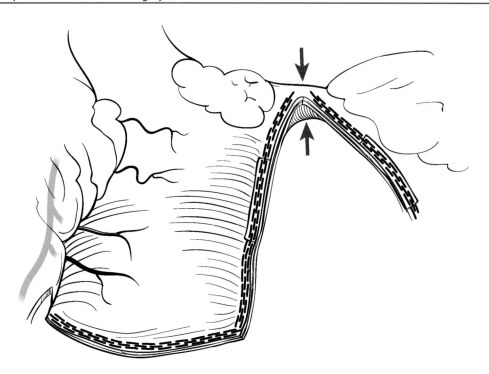

Fig. 14.20 The last firing of the top portion of the stomach often leaves an undivided 1–3 mm gastric portion. *Arrows* indicate the necessity of firing a final load beyond the visible staple line to avoid inadvertent opening leading to leaks

to the thickness of the stomach to avoid the disruption of the staple line. The Roux limb is then pulled up in an antecolic, antegastric fashion. Extreme attention must be paid not to twist the long Roux limb during this part of the operation. If the Roux limb looks short and the anastomosis is under tension, there are a few tricks to fix the problem. If the limb is still short, the patient should be placed back in the supine position, and the peritoneum covering the crotch of the divided mesentery should be opened. This will usually give enough length to relieve the tension. It is also possible to score the mesentery with the harmonic shears in a radiating fashion; this will ease the tension on the Roux-en-Y by lengthening it (Fig. 14.21). If the length is still insufficient, then one can divide the lesser omentum all the way up to the right crus of the diaphragm to release the attachments of the esophagus and add to the length of the pouch (Dr. Ninh Nguyen's technique, Fig. 14.22). Alternatively, the anastomosis can be performed in a retrocolic, retrogastric fashion, which traverses a shorter distance than the antecolic technique, but we have not needed to use this. The patient is then placed in reverse Trendelenberg position, and the gastro-jejunostomy is performed. The first posterior layer is sutured using a 3–0 Prolene on an SH1 starting in the first centimeter in the vertical division and finishing at the lesser curvature. This technique has dramatically reduced the number of postoperative strictures due to the creation of a larger anastomosis (Fig. 14.23). The enterotomy and gastrostomy are completed using the harmonic shears to a length of 1.5 cm (Figs. 14.24 and 14.25). If there is a little bleeding on the mucosa, it is possible to control it with intraluminal clips. Electrocautery should be avoided, as it can result in a postoperative leak (Fig. 14.26).

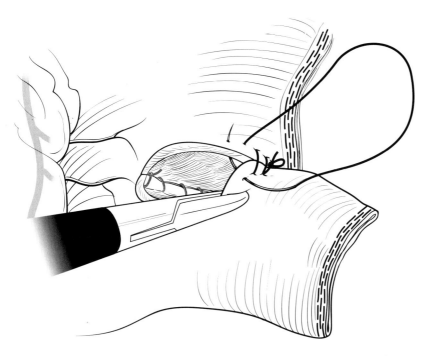

Fig. 14.28 Running the first anterior layer using an extramucosal 3–0 SH1 Prolene suture

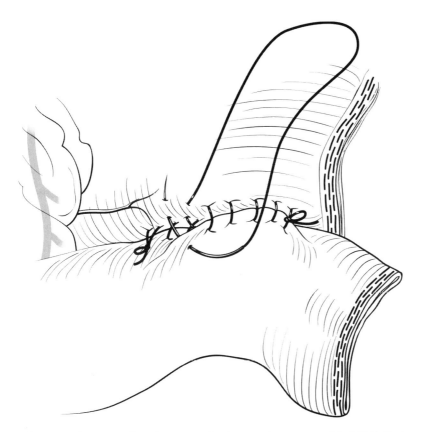

Fig. 14.29 Running the second and last anterior layer using a serosal 3–0 SH1 Prolene suture

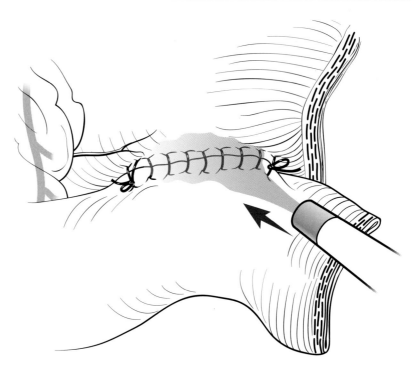

Fig. 14.30 Optional reinforcement of the anastomosis using fibrin glue

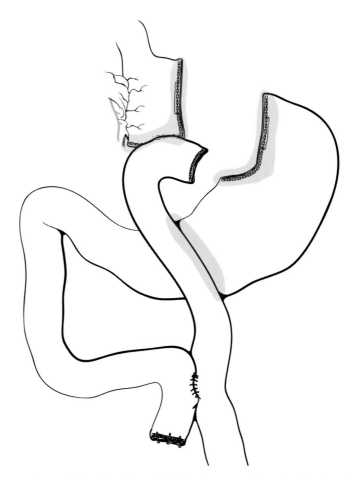

Fig. 14.31 Areas where fibrin glue is applied for hemostasis and adhesion (vertical gastric staple lines, Petersen's defect)

Immediate Postoperative Complications

There are two immediate postoperative complications for which patients may need to be emergently taken back to the operating room: bleeding and leak

■ **Bleeding.** In the immediate postoperative period, if a patient becomes tachycardic with a drop in the hemoglobin/hematocrit and sanginous fluid inside the drain, this is usually indicative of bleeding from the staple line. Most of the time, this is self-limited and responds to transfusion. However, if the patient continues to bleed and the drain keeps filling with blood, the surgeon should have a set point to take the patient back. In our experience, if the patient's hemoglobin drops below 8.5, or the hematocrit drops below 25 regardless of the vital signs, the patient should be taken back emergently to the operating room.

The abdomen is insufflated with a Veress needle. The same trocar incisions can be used, with the supraumbilical incision generally used to enter the abdomen. A large amount of clot may be seen around the bleeding area without any evidence of the bleeding vessel. Two other trocars are placed in a triangular fashion. The first step is to suck all the clots with a 10-mm suction catheter to clean the area. Introduction of a raytek can help accomplish this task. After the clots are removed, the area is thoroughly examined to find the bleeder, which will be clipped. After meticulous examination, the raytek is removed and another drain is placed. The application of fibrin sealant on all of the staple lines completes the procedure (Fig. 14.32).

Occasionally the bleeding is intraluminal. Intraoperative endoscopy will reveal if the bleeding is on the pouch side or the remnant side. If it is in the pouch, it can be controlled with endoscopic coagulation; however, if there is no blood inside the pouch, the source of bleeding must be the remnant. The solution is to oversew the staple line with a running suture.

■ **Leak.** In contrast to nonobese patients, tachycardia is the first and sometimes the only sign of a leak in obese patients. Any tachycardia above 100 beats/min is concerning and needs to be worked up. Our first step in work up is a stat CT scan with IV and oral contrast. In our experience, gastrographin swallow is not as sensitive as CT scan in detecting leaks, and the other benefit of CT scan is that it will detect other causes for tachycardia (i.e., fluid collections such as hematoma or rarely an abscess). Small leaks in stable patients can usually be managed with percutaneous drainage, antibiotics, and by keeping the patient NPO. Also, it may be possible to use intraluminal covered stents to traverse the leak. However, patients who become septic or rapidly fail nonoperative management need to be taken back promptly to the operating room.

After insufflation of the abdomen and placing the trocars in a triangular fashion, the area of leak is examined. If the leak is at the jejunojejunostomy, placement of extra sutures with an omental patch will often suffice. Otherwise, the anastomosis should be re-done. A leak at the gastrojejunostomy is usually not amenable to repair with suture due to severe inflammation from gastric secretions. Leak from this area is controlled with an omental patch and extensive drainage with multiple drains. Again, intraluminal stents maybe helpful if the leak is at the angle of His .

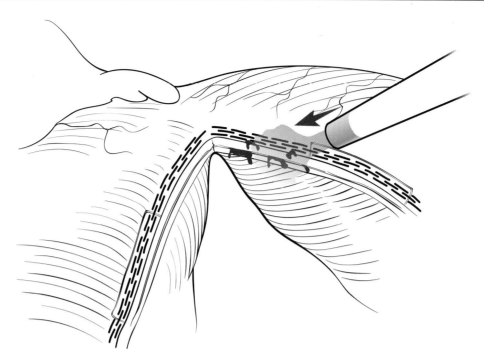

Fig. 14.32 Application of fibrin glue on bleeding staple lines

Late Postoperative Complications

Internal Hernia. Persistent colicky abdominal pain with vomiting in a patient after Roux-en-Y gastric bypass can be indicative of an internal hernia. Even if the mesenteric defect was closed in the original operation, it may enlarge as the patients lose weight and allow a loop of bowel to herniate (Fig. 14.33). The diagnostic tool of choice is a CT scan with IV and oral contrast, which will show a swirl of the mesenteric vessels around the internal hernia – the Cinnamon Roll sign. In this case, or if there is a high clinical suspicion for internal hernia, the patient should be taken back to the operating room. After insufflation and placement of a set of triangulated trocars, the ileal-cecal junction is found and bowel is run towards the ligament of Treitz. When the hernia is found, the small bowel is reduced and the mesenteric defect is closed with a nonabsorbable suture (Fig. 14.34). Fibrin sealant is applied over the defect (Fig. 14.35).

A grave complication is torsion of the small bowel, and more specifically torsion of the Roux limb. This is especially true with a long loop measuring more than 100 cm, as is the case in patients with a BMI greater than 50. When positioning the Roux-en-Y limb, it is possible to have a loose 360° torsion of the Roux limb, and the patient will present with multiple admissions to the ER with symptoms of vomiting and abdominal pain that resolve spontaneously. A contrast CT can be diagnostic, but more often, a diagnostic laparoscopy will find this rare complication. The only solution is to redo the gastrojejunostomy (Fig. 14.36).

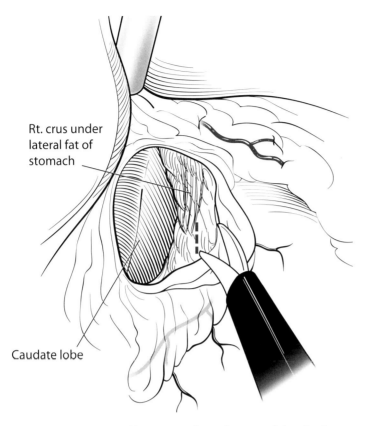

Fig. 14.39 Incision of the peritoneal layer over the right crus of the diaphragm

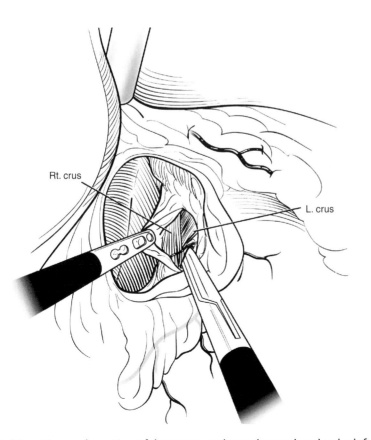

Fig. 14.40 Dissection and creation of the retroesophageal tunnel under the left crus, near the decussation of the crura

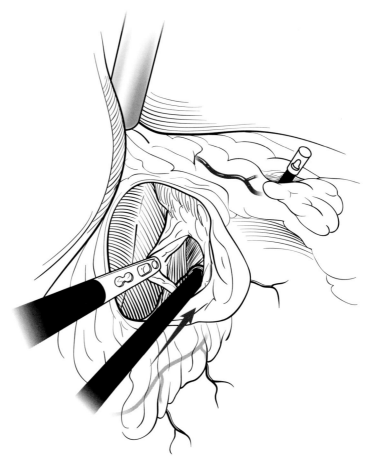

Fig. 14.41 The Goldfinger dissector is passed through the retroesophageal tunnel

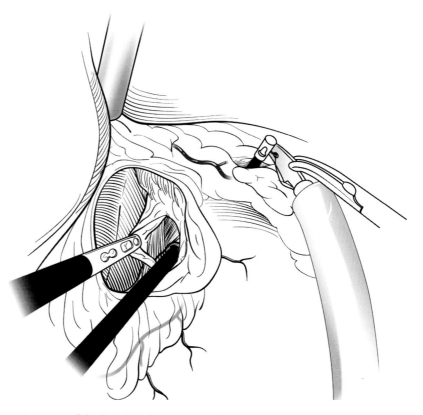

Fig. 14.42 Passage of the band in the retroesophageal tunnel

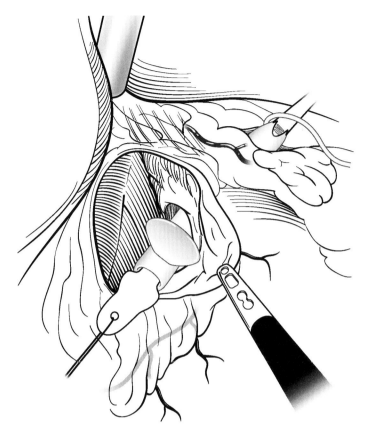

Fig. 14.43 Band placed according to the "Pars Flaccida" technique

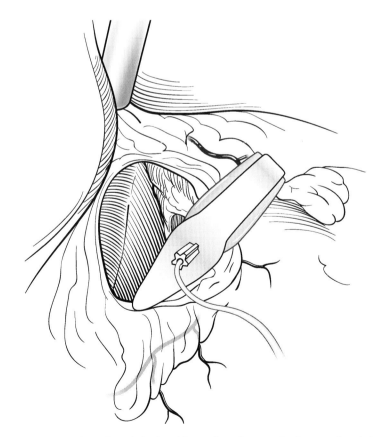

Fig. 14.44 The band is closed and the buckle is placed towards the caudate lobe of the liver, thus leaving the inflated chamber on the gastric wall

The first stitch attaches the stomach to the left crus (a French technique, Fig. 14.45) as an alternative to the gastric wall. Two other gastro-gastric stitches are placed to fix the band in the correct 45° position (Fig. 14.46). It is important that these stitches are placed high on the stomach to leave sufficient space for the Realize Band. A fourth stitch is used to reconstitute the phrenoesophageal membrane covering the right crus (Katkhouda stitch), and the last stitch is placed under the band itself, to further minimize the risk of slippage (Patterson's stitch). The last two stitches are optional. After this is done, the tubing is grasped and exteriorized through the 15 mm trocar. At this time, the incision of the fifteen millimeter trocar is widened to about 4 cm (Fig. 14.47), and a small area of the fascia is identified under the trocar entry site. A pocket is created, and the port-a-cath is fixed in place using a specially provided device (Fig. 14.48). It is important to ensure that the tubing is not twisted. We like to add a single vicryl stitch to approximate the fascia around the tubing to avoid any herniation. The subcutaneous fat and skin are closed in layers, and the remaining incisions are then closed using dermabond.

Complications

There are two major complications related to the lap band that would necessitate a revisional procedure: slippage and erosion.

■ **Slippage.** If the fundus is not plicated above the band, the stomach can slip under the band. If a patient continues to overeat in spite of having a very tight band, the pressure inside the pouch results in distention of the pouch. Over time, this excessive distention pushes the stomach through the band and results in slippage. On a plain X-ray of the abdomen, instead of appearing at a 45° angle pointing from the left shoulder to the right lower quadrant, the band will be in a horizontal plane or even at a 90° angle to the appropriate position (pointing from the right shoulder to the left lower quadrant).

The first step is to remove all the fluid from the band and keep the patient on liquid diet. This may result in reversal of the slipped pouch; however, if this maneuver is unsuccessful, the patient should be taken back to the operating room.

The positioning and trocar placement is exactly the same as the initial lap band operation. The adhesions of the liver to the band are taken down with harmonic shears. Then the gastro-gastric imbricating sutures are divided and the imbrication is reversed. Occasionally this can be done with an endo-GIA if the planes are obliterated. The band is then unlocked and removed, which results in release of the slippage. The options now are to make a new retroesophageal tract to place the same band, or preferably to convert the procedure to a Roux-en-Y gastric bypass (if discussed with the patient preoperatively).

■ **Erosion.** Erosions usually happen if the band is too tight or if there was an injury to the stomach in the original operation. Infection of the port site is commonly the first symptom of band erosion. It is diagnosed with endoscopy, which reveals a part of the band inside the stomach.

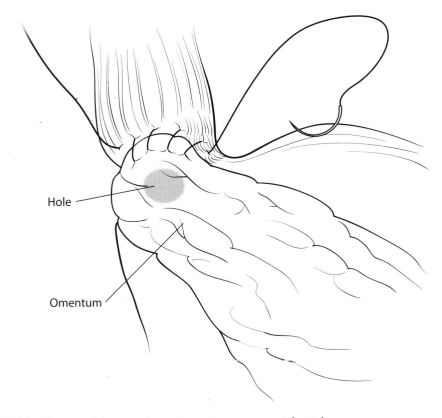

Fig. 14.52 Closure of the gastric erosion using an omental patch

The purpose is to create a 60–200 cc pouch removing a major part of the stomach, creating a sleeve and preserving a portion of the antrum (Fig. 14.53). The patient is placed in a steep reverse Trendelenburg position (Fig. 14.54). Good exposure of the stomach, by ensuring the stomach is stretched, is crucial for the dissection of the greater curvature. The harmonic shear is used to take down all the branches of the left gastroepiploic vessels. The greater curvature dissection continues approximately two centimeters to the pylorus, then a distance of five to six centimeters proximal to the pylorus is identified to start the first firing (Fig. 14.55). The sleeve gastrectomy is performed via sequential firings of a GIA forty-five starting with a 4.8 mm (green) stapler enforced with bioabsorbable material Seamguard (W.L. Gore Associates, Flagstaff AZ). The first stapler is fired so that a narrow 1.5 cm gap is left between the tip of the stapler and the lesser curvature (Fig. 14.56). The second firing is then performed, making sure that there is no occlusion of the gastric lumen. A 32–34, French bougie is then inserted and advanced along the lesser curvature into the duodenum to allow the calibration of the sleeve (Fig. 14.57) and then the sleeve gastrectomy, is completed by the firing of GIA-45 blue cartridges at the angle of His (Fig. 14.58). It is important to leave some gastric tissue at the upper edge near the angle of His to avoid injuring the gastro-esophagal junction. Seamguards are used on all firings. The gastric specimen is then removed through the umbilical port in a specimen bag (Fig. 14.59). An alternative technique is to divide the stomach before dividing the high gastroepiploic vessels and the short gastric vessels, thus allowing the stomach to remain attached and naturally retracted (Fig. 14.60). It is also possible to imbricate the areas of intersecting staple lines with interrupted stiches as an additional safety measure (Fig. 14.61).

Laparoscopic Sleeve Gastrectomy

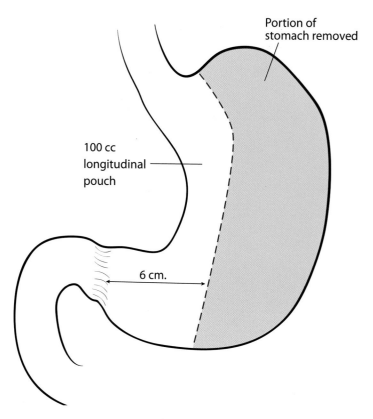

Fig. 14.53 Laparoscopic sleeve gastrectomy

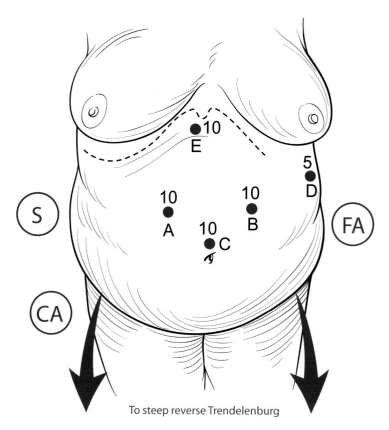

Fig. 14.54 Trocar port positions. *C* camera port; *A* left hand of surgeon; *B* right hand of surgeon; *D* grasper for assistant; *E* liver retractor

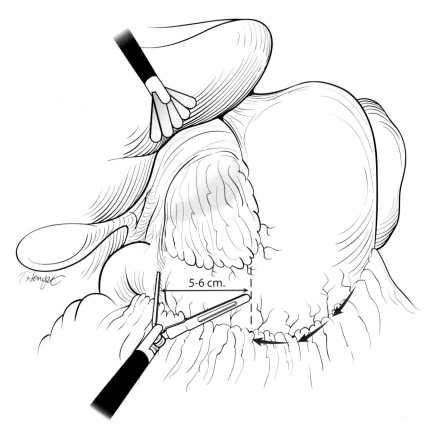

Fig. 14.55 Mobilization of the greater curvature to a distance of 5–6 cm of the pylorus

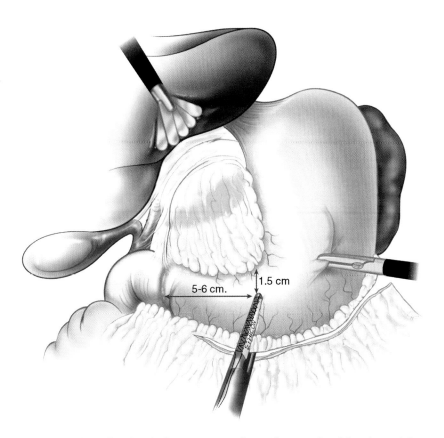

Fig. 14.56 Firing of the first load of a 45-mm stapler with green load, leaving a 1.5-cm margin to the lesser curve

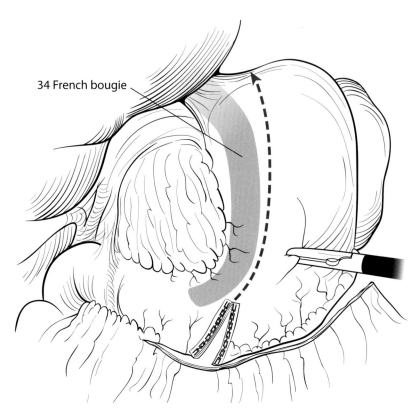

34 French bougie

Fig. 14.57 Introduction of a 34Fr bougie after the completion of the second firing of the stapler

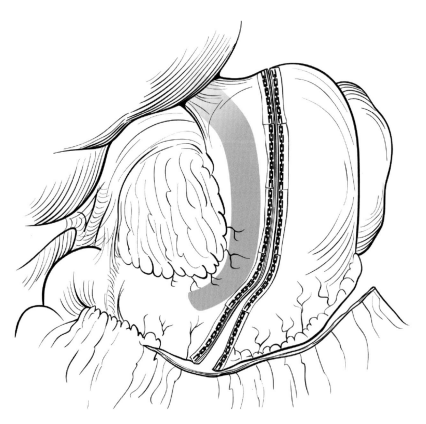

Fig. 14.58 Completion of the sleeve gastrectomy, all staple lines reinforced with Seamguard. Note that there is a sliver of stomach left at the angle of His to reduce the risk of postoperative leaks at this area

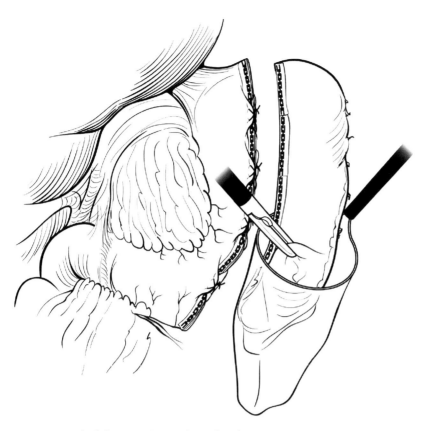

Fig. 14.59 Removal of the gastric specimen in a bag

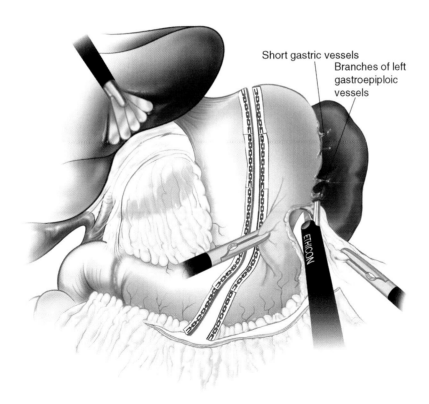

Short gastric vessels

Branches of left gastroepiploic vessels

Fig. 14.60 Alternative technique for sleeve gastrectomy. Mobilization of the greater curve and fundus following the division of the stomach, thus allowing for a natural retraction of the stomach during stapling

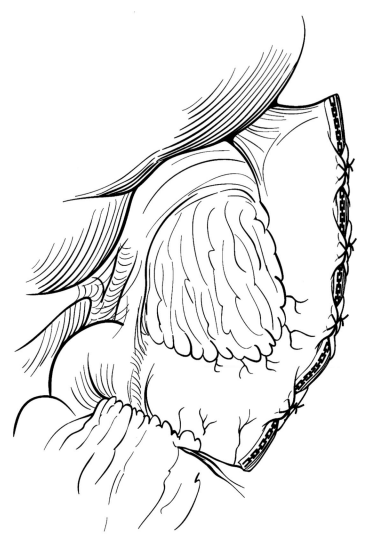

Fig. 14.61 Final view of the completed sleeve gastrectomy. The intersections of the staple lines are dunked using interrupted stitches

Arterburn D, Livingston EH, Schifftner T, Kahwati LC, Henderson WG, Maciejewski ML (2009) Predictors of long-term mortality after bariatric surgery performed in Veterans Affairs medical centers. Arch Surg 144(10):914–20

Collins BJ, Miyashita T, Schweitzer M, Magnuson T, Harmon JW (2007) Gastric bypass: why Roux-en-Y? A review of experimental data. Arch Surg 142(10):1000–1003; discussion 1004

Flum DR, Belle SH, King WC, Wahed AS, Berk P, Chapman W, Pories W, Courcoulas A, McCloskey C, Mitchell J, Patterson E, Pomp A, Staten MA, Yanovski SZ, Thirlby R, Wolfe B (2009) Perioperative safety in the longitudinal assessment of bariatric surgery. Longitudinal Assessment of Bariatric Surgery (LABS) Consortium. N Engl J Med 361(5):445–54

Frezza EE, Mammarappallil JG, Witt C, Wei C, Wachtel MS (2009) Value of routine post-operative gastrographin contrast swallow studies after laparoscopic gastric banding. Arch Surg 144(8):766–9

Higa KD, Boone KB, Ho T, Davies OG (2000) Laparoscopic Roux-en-Y gastric bypass for morbid obesity: technique and preliminary results of our first 400 patients. Arch Surg 135(9):1029–33

Katkhouda N, Moazzez A, Gondek S, Lam B (2008) A new and standardized technique for trocar placement in laparoscopic Gastric Bypass. Surg Endosc 23(3):659–62

Khoueir P, Black MH, Crookes PF, Kaufman H, Katkhouda N (2009) Way MY Prospective assesment of axial backpain symptoms before and after bariatric weightloss surgery. Spine J 9(6):454–63

Nguyen NT, Root J, Zainabadi K, Sabio A, Chalifoux S, Stevens CM, Mavandadi S, Longoria M, Wilson SE (2005) Accelerated growth of bariatric surgery with the introduction of minimally invasive surgery. Arch Surg 140(12):1198–202

Puzziferri N, Austrheim-Smith IT, Wolfe BM, Wilson SE, Nguyen NT (2006) Three-year follow-up of a prospective randomized trial comparing laparoscopic versus open gastric bypass. Ann Surg 243(2):181–8

Smith BR, Hinojosa MW, Reavis KM, Nguyen NT (2008) Remission of diabetes after laparoscopic gastric bypass. Ann Surg 74(10):948–52

Suter M, Calmes JM, Paroz A, Romy S, Giusti V (2009) Results of Roux-en-Y gastric bypass in morbidly obese vs superobese patients: similar body weight loss, correction of comorbidities, and improvement of quality of life. Arch Surg 144(4):312–8

Thodiyil PA, Yenumula P, Rogula T, Gorecki P, Fahoum B, Gourash W, Ramanathan R, Mattar SG, Shinde D, Arena VC, Wise L, Schauer P (2008) Selective nonoperative management of leaks after gastric bypass: lessons learned from 2675 consecutive patients. Ann Surg 248(5):782–92

**Selected
Further
Reading**

Single-Access Laparoscopic Surgery (SALS)

15

The concept of single-access laparoscopic surgery is to perform the procedure through one skin access (port). Several acronyms have been used to describe this concept, such as our single-access laparoscopic surgery (SALS), single port access (SPA) laparoendoscopic single-site surgery (LESS), and single incision laparoscopic surgery (SILS), and they all refer to the same procedure.

Basic Transumbilical Procedures

The umbilicus is usually used for basic procedures such as laparoscopic cholecystectomy, appendectomy, and hernias. The incision can circumscribe the umbilicus or go through the umbilicus, as depicted in Fig. 15.1. In the latter technique, the umbilicus is carefully cleaned, and two kocher clamps invert the umbilicus to expose the skin. An eleven blade is used to cut the skin, and then the skin incision is enlarged with a Kelly. Two S-retractors are inserted to retract the edges of the skin incision, and a fine scissor is used to create a pocket, developing a fascial plane slightly larger than the skin incision. It is then important to identify the natural defect in the linea alba, which is then enlarged by inserting a Kelly and spreading it open. Carefully, a blunt 5-mm trocar, preferably without any protuberant plastic edges, is inserted and the abdomen is then insufflated. At this point, a special long 40 cm, 5 mm, 30° bronchoscope (Karl Storz, Tuttlingen, Germany) is inserted between and hooked to the camera, and the exploration of the abdomen is performed. All the trocars are then inserted in a *staggered fashion* (Fig. 15.2). This figure also clearly shows the relationship of the different trocars and the long 5 mm scope. Ideally, they should be *short and stealthy* to avoid the "knitting needle" effect of the trocars. We prefer insertion of the 5 mm camera site at about 7 o'clock for a laparoscopic cholecystectomy, with one 5 mm trocar at 11 and one at 3 o'clock (Fig. 15.3) to allow the two hands to be positioned comfortably one on top of the other (Fig. 15.4). This describes the technique

N. Katkhouda, *Advanced Laparoscopic Surgery*,
DOI: 10.1007/978-3-540-74843-4_15, © Springer-Verlag Berlin Heidelberg 2011

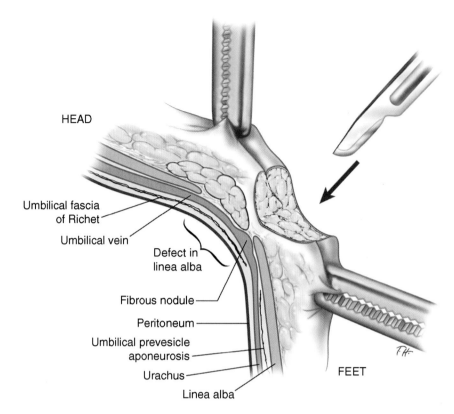

HEAD

Umbilical fascia
of Richet

Umbilical vein

Defect in
linea alba

Fibrous nodule

Peritoneum

Umbilical prevesicle
aponeurosis

Urachus

FEET

Linea alba

Fig. 15.1 Schematic view of the umbilicus; all the constituting layers are shown; two Kocher clamps evert the umbilical skin

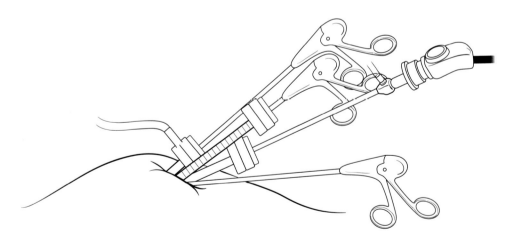

Fig. 15.2 Staggered insertion of trocars; use of a long 45 cm 5 mm 30° scope

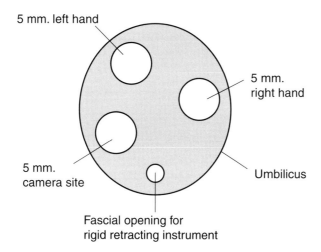

5 mm. left hand

5 mm.
right hand

5 mm.
camera site

Umbilicus

Fascial opening for
rigid retracting instrument

Fig. 15.3 Multiple fascial openings for SALS, all located within the umbilicus

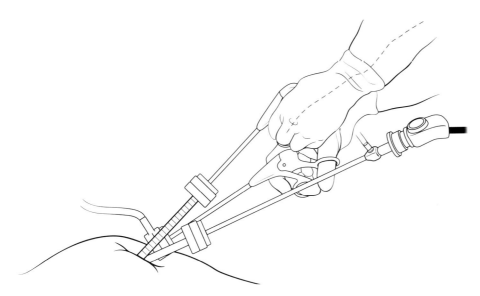

Fig. 15.4 Left operating hand supinated and positioned above pronated right hand of surgeon

using multiple small 5 mm facial openings under the divided skin of the umbilicus. One can also use disposable perforated rubber like devices offered by several companies that would require one slightly larger facial incision (around 2 cm).

The fundamental difference between SALS and classic laparoscopy is that the angle of the operation is much wider in the classic technique, therefore allowing a greater degree of freedom outside while the instruments are joining at the tips of the target. In SALS, because of the divergence that occurs early on at the skin level, the two tips reach the target at diverging angles (Fig. 15.5); as such, the only ways to allow for the right-hand instrument to reach the target are to cross the hands (Fig. 15.6) or to use the left hand as the dissecting hand, with the right hand as the supporting hand (Fig. 15.7). Again our solution is to avoid unnatural movements of the hands and keep them on top of each other thus allowing for more lateral freedom (Fig. 15.4).

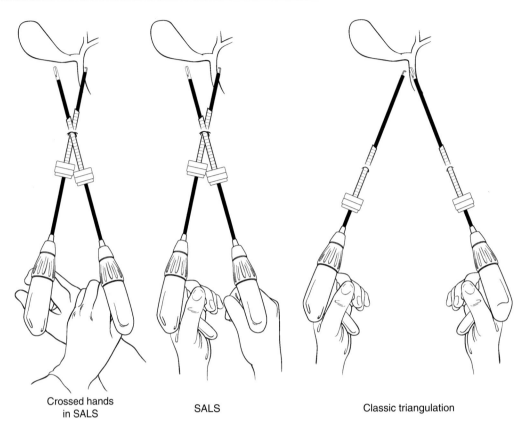

Crossed hands
in SALS

SALS

Classic triangulation

Fig. 15.5 Different angulation of instruments; classic triangulation during laparoscopy; SALS with and without crossing hands

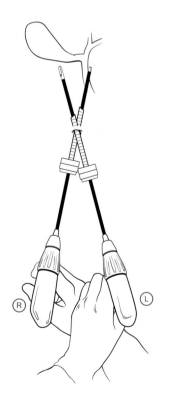

Fig. 15.6 Dissection of the cystic duct using a hook with the right hand crossed

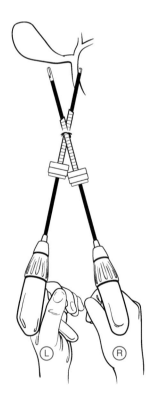

Fig. 15.7 Alternative technique: dissection of the cystic duct using a hook with the left hand

Advanced Laparoscopic Suturing Techniques

16

Laparoscopic suturing is a fundamental skill in advanced laparoscopic surgery. It requires a great deal of patience and practice. The mastery of this skill will enable the surgeon to perform many complex laparoscopic procedures and to laparoscopically repair complications should they occur.

Monitors

In performing complex laparoscopic surgery, the ergonomics of the operating room are of paramount importance. The monitor should be comfortably located at the level of surgeon's eyes, facing the surgeon on the side of the lesion. For example, during a cholecystectomy the monitor should be positioned on the patient's right side in direct line of vision of the surgeon. While during a laparoscopic Nissen the surgeon stands between the legs of the patient in the French position with the monitor placed at the head of the patient facing the surgeon.

OR Table

The height of the table should correspond to the surgeon's height, which will naturally place the surgeon's arms at the correct position to maneuver the laparoscopic instruments. The wrists should be straight, and the elbows comfortable. If the wrists are flexed (Fig. 16.1), either the table is too high or the trocars are placed too high. To fix a height discrepancy between the surgeon and the table, one should either readjust the table or use steps. If the problem is not fixed with adjustment of the table, the ports are placed too high and need to be repositioned to a lower location.

Ergonomics of the Operating Room (OR Table Height, Monitor Placement)

N. Katkhouda, *Advanced Laparoscopic Surgery*,
DOI: 10.1007/978-3-540-74843-4_16, © Springer-Verlag Berlin Heidelberg 2011

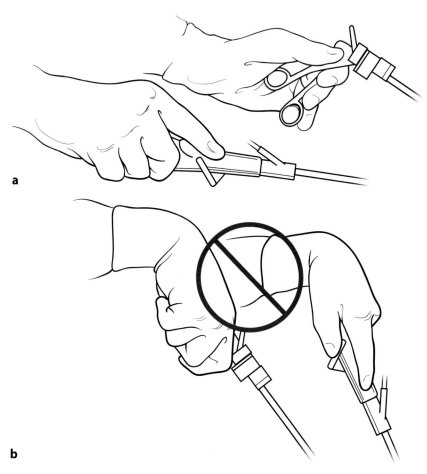

Fig. 16.1 Correct position of wrists. (**a**) depicts wrists in line with the forearms. (**b**) depicts incorrect flexed wrist position (operating table too high or trocar ports placed too high)

In addition, the table can be manipulated to the advantage of the surgeon. For example, during a laparoscopic appendectomy, tilting the table right side up and head down helps to move the small bowel into the left upper quadrant for better exposure. In essence, tilting the table creates an extra hand.

Trocar Placement and Triangulation

Successful laparoscopic suturing is dependent on a key concept in laparoscopic surgery, the *triangulation of instruments*. Triangulation occurs when the right and left hands of the surgeon are positioned on either side of the camera and form a 90° angle with the camera. This is the basic trocar position and will avoid the "knitting needle" effect of the instruments when using a two-handed technique. In addition to the triangulation of trocars at the skin at ninety degrees with the laparoscope, it is important to insert the trocar in such a way that the instruments also triangulate inside the abdomen at ninety degrees in a *double triangulation* (Fig. 1.11, Chap. 1). This is critical and especially important in patients who are morbidly obese with a thick abdominal wall. A trocar that is inserted straight down does not allow any movements of the instruments.

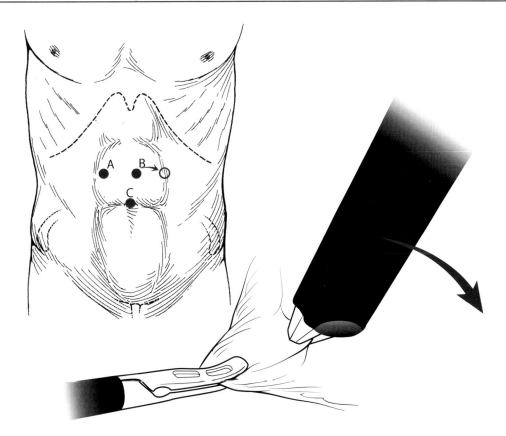

Fig. 16.2 "Shaft" sign; trocar for the surgeon's right hand is too medial. Tip of instrument is barely visible. The solution for this is lateral translation of the medialized port. *C* camera port; *A* left hand; *B* right hand, moved laterally

The intra-abdominal triangulation prevents the instruments from aligning themselves parallel to each other, which would make the task of suturing very difficult. Another common problem encountered in port placement is when a trocar is placed too medially and too close to the camera port. In this situation, instead of only visualizing the tip of the instrument in the field, the shaft is partially in line with the camera and will obstruct the view; this is known as the "shaft sign" (Fig. 16.2), and indicates an incorrect trocar position. The solution is to move the trocar by partially removing it and then sliding the skin with the help of the trocar more laterally before reinserting it.

The ideal ergonomic position for the camera is when the laparoscope is in line with the target while preserving the double triangulation. This ensures the optimal view required for successful laparoscopic suturing.

Equipment

Designated advanced laparoscopic equipment is necessary to perform advanced procedures. This equipment includes additional specifications for the purposes of laparoscopic suturing.

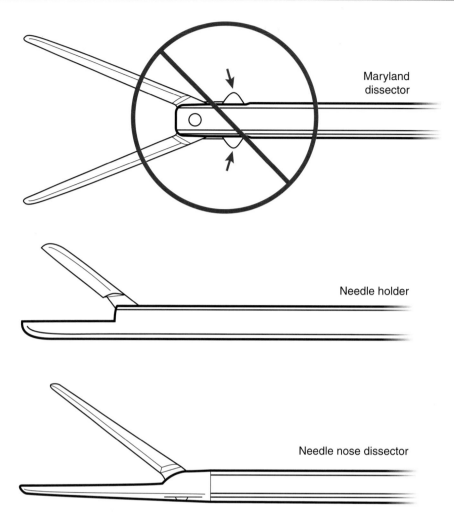

Fig. 16.3 Ideal instruments for laparoscopic suturing. Avoid exposed hinges associated with double action instruments. The best instruments are usually single-hinged. Needle nose grasper for the receiving and supporting hand is shown here

Needle Holders

Appropriate needle-holders are necessary, at least for the surgeon's dominant hand. The ideal needle-holder has a long shaft, a straight handle that allows some rotation of the wrist, and jaws with a diamond shape that will grasp the needle appropriately. The trigger mechanism of the needle-holder should be comfortable, and the jaws should grasp firmly enough without use of excessive force, which may crush and break the suture. The needle-holder should be single action without any exposed hinges in which the suture material can be caught (Fig. 16.3).

Graspers

Graspers should be atraumatic and without ratchets. Fenestration is a matter of surgeon's preference. The only grasper with a ratchet is used to retract the gallbladder during a cholecystectomy. It is important to avoid graspers with exposed hinges in laparoscopic surgery, because the suture can become caught in the hinge during laparoscopic knot-tying. Most double action graspers are double-hinged; hence the author recommends use of single action grasper (needle nose grasper). The nondominant, supporting hand of the surgeon should ideally hold long, atraumatic, single-hinged forceps with jaws, without groove marks that would entrap the suture (Fig. 16.3).

Suture Material

Suture material choice is similar as in open surgery, however the rule is to use one "0" thicker than would be used in open surgery. Hence, 2–0 sutures should be used for the various muscular and fascial closures, and 3–0 sutures reserved for fine suturing such as on the esophagus, stomach or colon. Suture length is of paramount importance – 14 cm (6 in.) is sufficient for a single intra-abdominal knotted tie, 24 cm will suffice for a running suture, and a 90 cm (35 in.) thread is ideal for extracorporeal knot-tying. Shorter sutures will render the technique of intra and extracorporeal knot-tying more difficult and a frustrating struggle will ensue. Though there is no general rule, the author's preferred stitches would probably be a 3–0 Prolene on an SH1 needle (which is smaller than a regular SH) for suturing intra-abdominal organs, and a 2–0 Ethibond on an SH1 needle for muscular structures, such as the crura of the diaphragm.

Interrupted Stitch

The scrub technician prepares the thread by removing the memory and cutting the thread at the appropriate length: 14 cm for one interrupted stitch, 24 cm for a running stitch. The thread is grasped at least 5 mm from the needle and then the needle is introduced through the 10 mm port. As a policy, every time a needle is introduced into or taken out of the abdominal cavity, the surgeon will inform the circulating nurse to document it on the OR board. This prevents the future confusion of having a needle inside the abdominal cavity in case the needle count is incorrect.

As in open surgery, the needle is grasped one-third of the distance from the insertion of the thread to the tip. The movements of the hands should be natural, with the needle at 90° to the shaft of the needle-holder. The left hand grasps the tissue and presents it to the needle-holder as in open surgery, and usually once the needle has passed the first layer, it can be grabbed with the left hand and presented to the empty needle-holder again before entering the second, opposite layer.

A general principle of intracorporeal knot-tying is that the needle should always "smile" at the surgeon, and the tip of the needle should be at the Side of The Loose End of the thread ("STLE"). In other words, the thread should create an inverted "C" with the loop facing upwards (Fig. 16.4). With the loose end on the right side of the surgeon, the surgeon rotates the needle-holder (pronation of the wrist), advances the needle-holder on top of the grasper, rotates the needle-holder (supination of the wrist), and pulls the needle-holder back, all while the grasper remains unmoving. The tip of the grasper is then opened; the suture is grasped and pulled through to complete the knot. The opposite maneuver is made when the loose end is on the left side of the surgeon

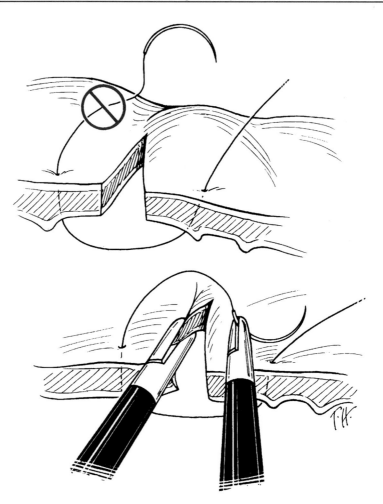

Fig. 16.4 The *bottom picture* illustrates the correct principle of intra-abdominal knotting. The needle "smiles" at the surgeon, and the tip of the needle should be on the side of the loose end ("STLE")

(Fig. 16.5 a, b). It is also important that the tips of the needle-holder and the grasper do not touch each other, as it will decrease the speed of suturing.

In summary, intracorporeal knotting resembles open microsurgical instrumental knot-tying. In the case of a surgeon who is left handed, the initial steps and the first square knot are achieved in the reverse position.

Running Stitch

Tying an intracorporeal knot after a running stitch follows the same principles as an interrupted stitch. It is important to use the correct suture length (24 cm for a running stitch). To retrieve the needle once the knot has been tied, the thread should be held very close to needle and gently pulled out through the port. If no thread remains, align the needle with the needle-holder and pull the needle out under direct vision of the camera.

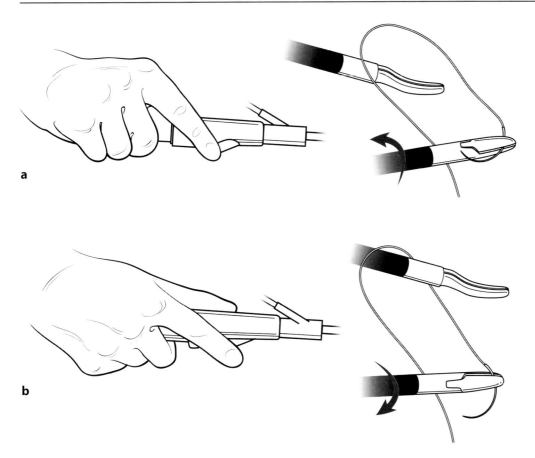

Fig. 16.5 (**a**) First throw and creation of the knot. (**b**) The suture is looped up to create a virtual suture omega Ω

Pirouette

The pirouette is a simple, elegant maneuver to position the needle on the needle-holder in an efficient manner. In this maneuver, the thread is grasped and used to pirouette the needle into place (Fig. 16.6). Once the needle is in the correct alignment, it can be simply grasped by the needle-holder if needed. This avoids the often clumsy, time consuming transfer of the needle between instruments, further dulling the needle and deforming the shape.

It is difficult to achieve high precision knot-tying using extracorporeal knot-tying. The author prefers to reserve extracorporeal knot-tying for suturing on the bone or muscle. For example, the crura of the diaphragm, the abdominal wall, and Cooper's ligament are all amenable to extracorporeal knot-tying.

Various knots are possible, but the two most popular techniques are (a) the creation of an external half-knot that is pushed by a knot pusher (Fig. 16.7), and (b) construction of Roeder's knot that is pushed inside using an atraumatic grasper (Fig. 16.8). It is advisable to leave long branches after cutting the ends of the knot – enough to be able to add an extra intra-abdominal knot to secure the other knots if necessary. This is achieved by using a thread of at least 90 cm (35 in.).

Extracorporeal Knot-Tying

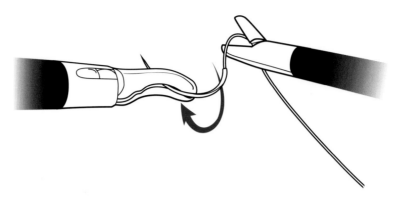

Fig. 16.6 "Pirouette"; the needle is maneuvered into the proper position with a rotation of the thread by the needle-holder, while the needle nose grasper loosely holds the needle itself

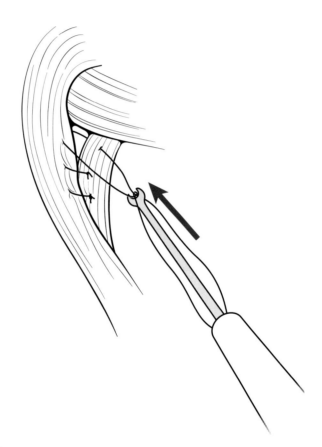

Fig. 16.7 Use of an extracorporeal knot pusher for closure of muscular tissues (crura shown here)

Roeder's Knot

Roeder's knot is similar to the concept of an Endoloop (Fig. 16.8). Half of a knot is tied, one of the suture tails is rotated three times around both threads, and then the same tail is introduced inside the gap formed by the original half-knot and the first rotation. The tail is then pulled through thus creating a sliding knot.

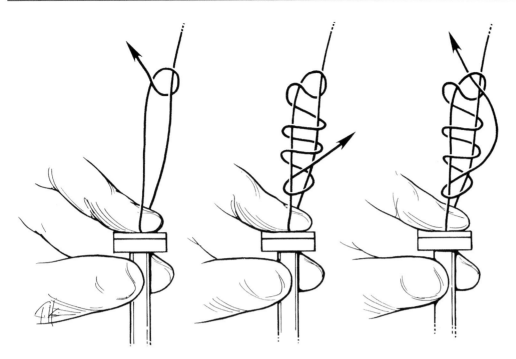

Fig. 16.8 Roeder's knot for extracorporeal knot-tying, using a 35-in. (90 cm) thread

Endoloop

It is also possible to use preformed knots such as Endoloops. The way to secure an Endoloop is to make sure that the organ to be knotted in the endoloop is free at one end, and then to pull it inside the loop with a grasper (Fig. 16.9).

One trick to avoid tearing the tissue is to place the grasper within the abdominal cavity to create a pulley effect, placing tension on the suture and not on the tissue. Next, bring the needle out, tie a knot and use the knot pusher to push the knot into the abdomen.

Lost Needle

If the needle is lost, do not move or insert any instruments. First, one should look inside the trocar as the needle may be caught within the shaft of the trocar. Then the scope is moved from the main trocar and placed into the working trocar to look for the needle. Next, one should examine the abdominal cavity without manipulating any tissue. The needle may be *floating on the fat* (Fig. 16.10 *1, 2, 3*). Once the tissue has been moved, the needle can slide into the tissue and sometimes may even be impossible to find, even requiring conversion to an open operation.

Short Suture

If the thread is very short and a critical suture has been placed and cannot be redone, the needle can be used to increase the length of the thread. Again, the needle should be in the smiling position, keeping the loose end on the side of the needle (STLE: The tip of the needle has to be on the side of the loose end), and otherwise using the same movements as in intracorporeal knot-tying to complete the knot.

Trouble-shooting

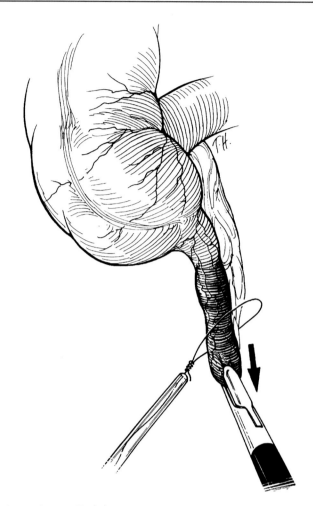

Fig. 16.9 Knot-tying using an Endoloop suture

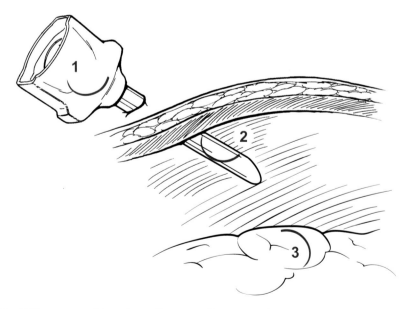

Fig. 16.10 Different usual location of lost needles: *1* needle located in the base of the trocar; *2* needle in trocar sleeve; *3* needle just located "floating" on fat, near the intra-abdominal tip of the trocar

Aggarwal R, Hance J, Undre S, Ratnasothy J, Moorthy K, Chang A, Darzi A (2006) Training junior operative residents in laparoscopic suturing skills is feasible and efficacious. Surgery 139(6):729–734

Ahmed S, Hanna GB, Cuschieri A (2004) Optimal angle between instrument shaft and handle for laparoscopic bowel suturing. Arch Surg 139(1):89–92

Facchin M, Bessell JR, Maddern GJ (1994) A simplified technique for laparoscopic instrument ties. Aust NZ J Surg 64(8):569–71

Fried GM, Feldman LS, Vassiliou MC, Fraser SA, Stanbridge D, Ghitulescu G, Andrew CG (2004) Proving the value of simulation in laparoscopic surgery. Ann Surg 240(3):518–25

Garcia-Ruiz A, Gagner M, Miller JH, Steiner CP, Hahn JF (1998) Manual vs robotically assisted laparoscopic surgery in the performance of basic manipulation and suturing tasks. Arch Surg 133(9):957–61

Jamshidi R, LaMasters T, Eisenberg D, Duh QY, Curet M (2009) Video self-assessment augments development of videoscopic suturing skill. J Am Coll Surg 209(5):622–5

Mackay S, Datta V, Chang A, Shah J, Kneebone R, Darzi A (2003) Multiple Objective Measures of Skill (MOMS): a new approach to the assessment of technical ability in surgical trainees. Ann Surg 238(2):291–300

Madan AK, Harper JL, Taddeucci RJ, Tichansky DS (2008) Goal-directed laparoscopic training leads to better laparoscopic skill acquisition. Surgery 144(2):345–50

McDougall EM, Kolla SB, Santos RT, Gan JM, Box GN, Louie MK, Gamboa AJ, Kaplan AG, Moskowitz RM, Andrade LA, Skarecky DW, Osann KE, Clayman RV (2009) Preliminary study of virtual reality and model simulation for learning laparoscopic suturing skills. J Urol 182(3):1018–25

Rosser JC, Rosser LE, Savalgi RS (1997) Skill acquisition and assessment for laparoscopic surgery. Arch Surg 132(2):200–4

Rosser JC Jr, Rosser LE, Savalgi RS (1998) Objective evaluation of a laparoscopic surgical skill program for residents and senior surgeons. Arch Surg 133(6):657–61

Ruiz de Adana JC, Hernández Matías A, Hernández Bartolomé M, Manzanedo Romero I, Leon Ledesma R, Valle Rubio A, López Herrero J, Limones Esteban M (2009) Risk of gastrojejunal anastomotic stricture with multifilament and monofilament sutures after hand-sewn laparoscopic gastric bypass: a prospective cohort study. Obes Surg 19(9):1274–1277

Schwarz RE, Julian TB (1995) A simple way to finish a continuous laparoscopic suture. Surg Endosc 9(5):547–548

Shatz DV, Block EJ, Kligman M (1994) Laparoscopic suturing technique for enteral access procedures. Surg Endosc 8(6):717–718

Wattanasirichaigoon S (1997) Triple-loop knot for securing a running suture in laparoscopic surgery. Br J Surg 84(3):422

Subject Index

hemigastrectomy 103
hemoglobin 235
Hemophilus influenza 181
   vaccination 181
hemorrhage 17, 22, 35, 62, 208, 210
hemostasis 15, 17, 35, 49, 55, 62, 69, 80, 93,
      106, 153, 190, 193, 195, 196, 200, 203,
      208, 226
hemostatic pad 29
hepatectomy 61
hepatic
   artery 45
   branch 71
   duct 25, 29, 33, 46, 261
      visual cholangiogram 33
   flexure 134
   lesion 50
   metastases 55
   parenchyma 55, 57
   resection 49
   surgery 50
   vascular isolation 58
   vein 53, 55, 58, 60, 62, 206, 209, 210
hepaticojejunostomy 44
hernia 86, 153, 163, 169, 257
   defect 155, 172, 174
      measurement 172
      size 172
   incisional 169, 177
   indirect 162
   procedure 9
   repair 7
   sac 86, 153, 155, 164
   ventral 169, 177
herniation 10, 244
hiatus 68–70, 89, 103, 239
   access 71
   area 80
   hernia 67
hilar
   artery 190
   vein 190
   vessel 13, 182, 187, 188, 190, 193
      maneuver of last resort 195
hilum 190, 195
hook 27
hydrodissection 18, 22, 181
hydroirrigation 28
hydrops 29
hypochondrium 8, 80

I
idiopathic thrombocytopenic purpura
      (ITP) 181
ileocolic vessel 133
ileus 143
iliac
   crest 203
   vein 149
      fluttering 164
   vessel 153, 155

iliopubic tract 149, 151, 153, 158, 160
incisional hernia 177
inferior
   epigastric vessel 149, 164
   phrenic vein 206
   pole vessel 190, 193, 196
   vena cava 49, 206, 208–210
inguinal
   canal 165
   hernia
      direct 149
      indirect 149
      repair 261
inguino-scrotal hernia 153
injury 25
   of superficial vessel 10
instruments 2, 9
   basic set 2
insufflation 14, 86, 139, 143, 186
   pressure 110
insufflator 15
intercostal nerve 177
   entrapment 177
   injury 177
internal
   hernia 220, 236
   oblique muscle 162, 178
intraabdominal
   abscess 125
   fat 13, 215
   pressure 143
intracorporeal
   knot-tying 58, 79
   suturing 29
intraluminal clip 228
intraoperative cholangiogram 41
intraperitoneal space 12
intraumbilical insertion 262
inverted Y position 3
irrigation/suction device 17, 18, 22, 29, 35,
      112, 181, 186
ischemia 71, 96, 239

J
jejunal loop 45, 107, 109, 219
jejunojejunostomy 46, 215, 220, 235

K
Kaiser stitch 220
Katkhouda stitch 244
Keith needle 261
Kelly
   clamp 17, 195, 257
   forceps 53, 55
keyhole slot 155
kidney 205
   superior pole 208
knitting needle effect 22, 50, 119, 257, 266